1st EDITION

Perspectives on Diseases and Disorders

Skin Cancer

Carrie Fredericks

Book Editor

PERSPECTIVES
On Diseases & Disorders

GALE
CENGAGE Learning™

Detroit • New York • San Francisco • New Haven, Conn • Waterville, Maine • London

GALE
CENGAGE Learning™

Christine Nasso, *Publisher*
Elizabeth Des Chenes, *Managing Editor*

For more information, contact:
Greenhaven Press
27500 Drake Rd.
Farmington Hills, MI 48331-3535
Or you can visit our Internet site at gale.cengage.com

Articles in Greenhaven Press anthologies are often edited for length to meet page requirements. In addition, original titles of these works are changed to clearly present the main thesis and to explicitly indicate the author's opinion. Every effort is made to ensure that Greenhaven Press accurately reflects the original intent of the authors. Every effort has been made to trace the owners of copyrighted material.

LIBRARY OF CONGRESS CATALOGING-IN-PUBLICATION DATA

Skin cancer / Carrie Fredericks, book editor.
p. cm. -- (Perspectives on diseases and disorders)
Includes bibliographical references and index.
ISBN 978-0-7377-4792-8 (hardcover)
1. Skin--Cancer. I. Fredericks, Carrie.
RC280.S5S5515 2010
616.99'477--dc22

2009048145

Printed in the United States of America
1 2 3 4 5 6 7 14 13 12 11 10

CONTENTS

FOREWORD

"Medicine, to produce health, has to examine disease."
—Plutarch

Independent research on a health issue is often the first step to complement discussions with a physician. But locating accurate, well-organized, understandable medical information can be a challenge. A simple Internet search on terms such as "cancer" or "diabetes," for example, returns an intimidating number of results. Sifting through the results can be daunting, particularly when some of the information is inconsistent or even contradictory. The Greenhaven Press series Perspectives on Diseases and Disorders offers a solution to the often overwhelming nature of researching diseases and disorders.

From the clinical to the personal, titles in the Perspectives on Diseases and Disorders series provide students and other researchers with authoritative, accessible information in unique anthologies that include basic information about the disease or disorder, controversial aspects of diagnosis and treatment, and first-person accounts of those impacted by the disease. The result is a well-rounded combination of primary and secondary sources that, together, provide the reader with a better understanding of the disease or disorder.

Each volume in Perspectives on Diseases and Disorders explores a particular disease or disorder in detail. Material for each volume is carefully selected from a wide range of sources, including encyclopedias, journals, newspapers, nonfiction books, speeches, government documents, pamphlets, organization newsletters, and position papers. Articles in the first chapter provide an authoritative, up-to-date overview that covers symptoms, causes and effects, treatments, cures, and medical advances. The second chapter presents a substantial number of opposing viewpoints on controversial treatments and other current debates relating to the volume topic. The third chapter offers a variety of personal perspectives on the disease or disorder. Patients, doctors, caregivers, and loved ones represent just some of the voices found in this narrative chapter.

Each Perspectives on Diseases and Disorders volume also includes:

- An **annotated table of contents** that provides a brief summary of each article in the volume.
- An **introduction** specific to the volume topic.
- Full-color **charts and graphs** to illustrate key points, concepts, and theories.
- Full-color **photos** that show aspects of the disease or disorder and enhance textual material.
- **"Fast Facts"** that highlight pertinent additional statistics and surprising points.
- A **glossary** providing users with definitions of important terms.
- A **chronology** of important dates relating to the disease or disorder.
- An annotated list of **organizations to contact** for students and other readers seeking additional information.
- A **bibliography** of additional books and periodicals for further research.
- A detailed **subject index** that allows readers to quickly find the information they need.

Whether a student researching a disorder, a patient recently diagnosed with a disease, or an individual who simply wants to learn more about a particular disease or disorder, a reader who turns to Perspectives on Diseases and Disorders will find a wealth of information in each volume that offers not only basic information, but also vigorous debate from multiple perspectives.

INTRODUCTION

Sunscreen is defined as a substance that protects the skin from excessive exposure to the sun's ultraviolet (UV) radiation. The first sunscreen was introduced in the United States in 1928, and since then different formulas and preparations have abounded. In 1978 the U.S. Food and Drug Administration (FDA) first proposed new safety regulations regarding sunscreens. Since then sunscreen rules have been proposed and changed several times. In 1997 Congress mandated that the FDA regulate sunscreen as an over-the-counter medication for the treatment and prevention of sunburn. This led to rules for protection

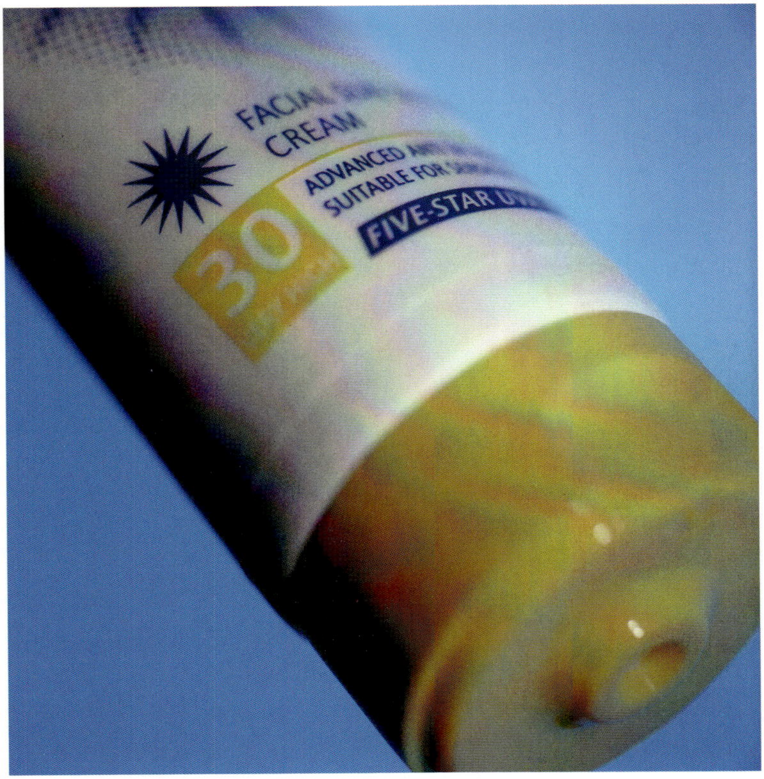

In 1997 the U.S. Congress mandated that the Food and Drug Administration regulate over-the-counter sunscreen for the prevention of sunburn. (**Steve Horrell/Photo Researchers, Inc.**)

from UVB rays, which cause cancer. In 2007 the FDA proposed additional rules, but this time those regulations included stipulations for UVA rays and standardized testing of all sunscreen formulas. After this proposal the FDA began to solicit opinions on the veracity of its rule changes. Sunscreens and the blocking of UV rays is becoming a more complicated issue; while the federal government and most medical professionals believe that sunscreens help immensely in the fight against skin cancer, there is a faction of health professionals that believes the sunscreen preparations themselves can cause cancer.

In 1972 the FDA had changed the classification of sunscreens from cosmetics to over-the-counter drug preparations. This allowed the FDA to propose rules for the use and labeling of these creams and lotions. During the next two decades, many suntan lotions and oils that contained no sunscreen ingredients whatsoever were being used as sun protection. In 1999 the FDA ruled that all suntan products that did not contain any sunscreen elements had to carry a warning label: "Warning—this product does not contain a sunscreen and does not protect against sunburn. Repeated exposure of unprotected skin while tanning may increase the risk of skin aging, skin cancer, and other harmful effects to the skin even if you do not burn."[1] This labeling, intended to help consumers be aware of the differences between suntan lotion and sunscreen, became effective in 2000.

Sunscreens can be effective against two different types of UV radiation: UVA and UVB. UVA radiation is the longest wavelength of the UV radiations and can penetrate more deeply into the skin. UVB rays have a shorter wavelength and are not as constant as UVA rays. The sun protection factor, or SPF, rating system is based on UVB rays. According to the Skin Cancer Foundation, "SPF numbers indicate how long it will take for UVB rays to redden your skin when you use a sun protection product, compared to how long the skin would take to redden without the product. The higher the SPF, the longer skin can be sun-exposed before burning."[2]

In 2007 the FDA expanded its sunscreen regulation proposal to include labeling that indicates the amount of protection offered against UVA rays. The new system will use a four-star rating alongside the current SPF rating. According to the FDA, the UVA rating system is designed as follows: "One star will represent low UVA protection; two stars, medium protection; three stars, high protection; four stars, the highest UVA protection available in an over-the-counter (OTC) sunscreen product. If a sunscreen product does not rate at least one star, FDA is proposing that its labeling bear a 'no UVA protection' marking on the front label near the SPF value."[3] These ratings would be based on a new standardized testing method. According to the Skin Cancer Foundation:

> The FDA rating would be based on two tests: the first, conducted in a lab (in vitro testing), would use a sun simulator to measure the "product's ability to reduce the amount of UVA radiation that passes through it." It would include a measurement for "photostability"—the sunscreen's ability to maintain effectiveness for some hours without being degraded by the sun. The second test, similar to the SPF test, would assess the sunscreen's ability to prevent tanning or reddening on a person (in vivo testing).[4]

In addition to the UVA ratings, the proposed rules are also looking at changing the maximum SPF number from 30 to 50. This SPF number of 50 would be the maximum sun protection factor that a company could claim its products contain. The FDA is also considering changing the terms used to describe UVB protection to low and medium instead of minimal and moderate. More changes include a warning box on the product label about the dangers of sun exposure and the risks of skin cancer: "UV exposure from the sun increases the risk of skin cancer, premature skin aging, and other skin damage. It is important to decrease the UV exposure by limiting the time in the sun, wearing protective clothing, and using a sunscreen."[5]

While waiting to implement these new regulations, the FDA has solicited comments from the public regarding these changes. More than twenty thousand comments and opinions were received regarding this issue. On the Web site TheHill.com, a political news and information site, physician Sandra Read weighs in and talks about the need to implement these new rules quickly. She says that the newest sunscreens with higher levels of UVA and UVB protection could be four times more effective in the prevention of melanoma than earlier sunscreens containing only UVB ingredients. "In my practice, I diagnose and treat the deadly effects of skin cancer every day. Enactment of a robust UVA standard and approval of the best sunscreen actives will offer the American public more tools to prevent this costly disease. It's time Americans have the same protection against the sun's harmful rays available in every other country for years."[6]

While the FDA sifts through the comments concerning the new regulations, some individuals in the medical community contend that sunscreen itself may cause cancer. Al Sears, an alternative medicine and anti-aging specialist, states that several very common sunscreen ingredients have dangerous and cancer-causing side effects. According to Sears, "Oxybenzone, sometimes called Benzophenone-3, is linked to allergies, hormone disruption, low birth weights, cell damage, and more. It also helps other chemicals penetrate the skin. . . . Octyl methoxycinnamate (OMC) kills skin cells. PABA, also known as octyl-dimethyl and padimate-O, attacks DNA and causes genetic mutation when it is exposed to sunlight."[7] To counteract sun damage, Sears recommends getting plenty of antioxidants, getting enough omega-3 fatty acids, and using mango or shea butter as a sun blocker.

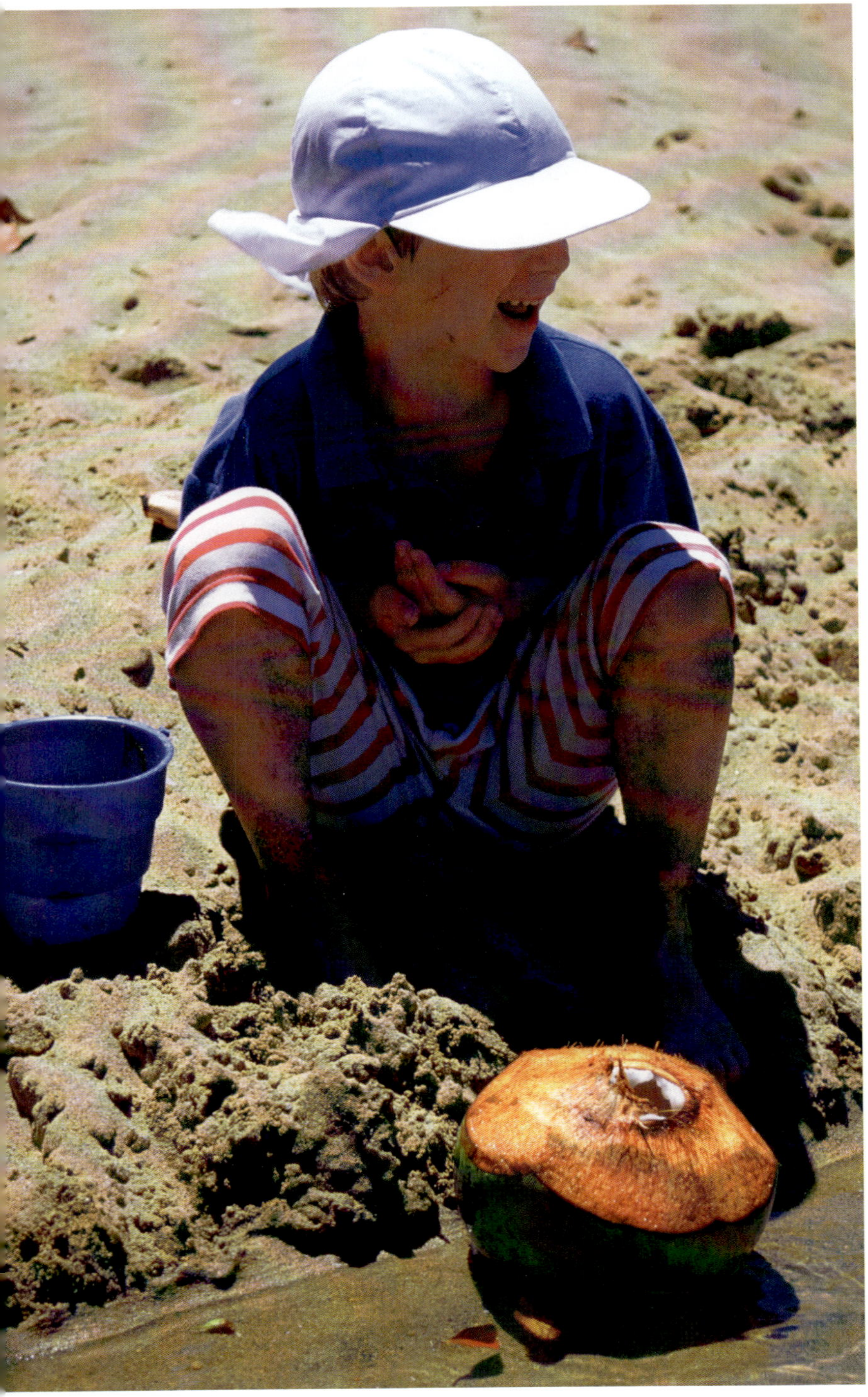

To help prevent skin cancer it is important to limit time spent in the sun, to wear protective clothing, and to use sunscreen. (© **Nick Hanna/Alamy**)

The evidence that sun exposure causes skin damage and can lead to skin cancer is overwhelming, but some, such as Sears, still contend that the sunscreens themselves are as dangerous as the sun's rays. The vast majority of physicians, however, do recommend daily use of sunscreen to avoid overexposure to the sun, which may lead to skin cancer. Over the last twenty years, the FDA has been discussing the implementation of new and improved sunscreen rules. These rules, covering UVA ratings, SPF ratings, sun exposure, and sun damage, are still under review. The nature of sunscreens has improved dramatically over this time period, and the FDA is hoping to make easier the process of choosing to protect oneself against sun damage.

1. U.S. Food and Drug Administration, "Required Warning Statement for Tanning Products Without Sunscreen," 2000. www.fda.gov/Cosmetics.

2. Skin Cancer Foundation, "FDA Proposes New Rules Mandating UVA Protection Labeling," 2007. www.skincancer.org.

3. U.S. Food and Drug Administration, "FDA Aims to Upgrade Sunscreen Labeling," August 23, 2007. www.fda.gov/ForConsumers/ConsumerUpdates/ucm 049091.htm.

4. Skin Cancer Foundation, "FDA Proposes New Rules Mandating UVA Protection Labeling," 2007. www.skincancer.org.

5. Quoted in Riette van Laack, "FDA Proposes Monograph for OTC Sunscreens Addressing Protection Against UVA and UVB Light," FDA Law Blog, August 29, 2007. www.fdalawblog.net/fda_law_blog_hyman_phelps/2007/08/fda-proposes-mo.html.

6. Sandra Read, "FDA Should Test Sunscreens' Effectiveness vs. Skin Cancer," The Hill, July 20, 2009. http://thehill.com/letters.

7. Al Sears, "Avoid This Cancer-Causing Trap," Power for Healthy Living, 2009. www.alsearsmd.com/prevent-skin-cancer.html.

CHAPTER 1

Overview: Understanding Skin Cancer

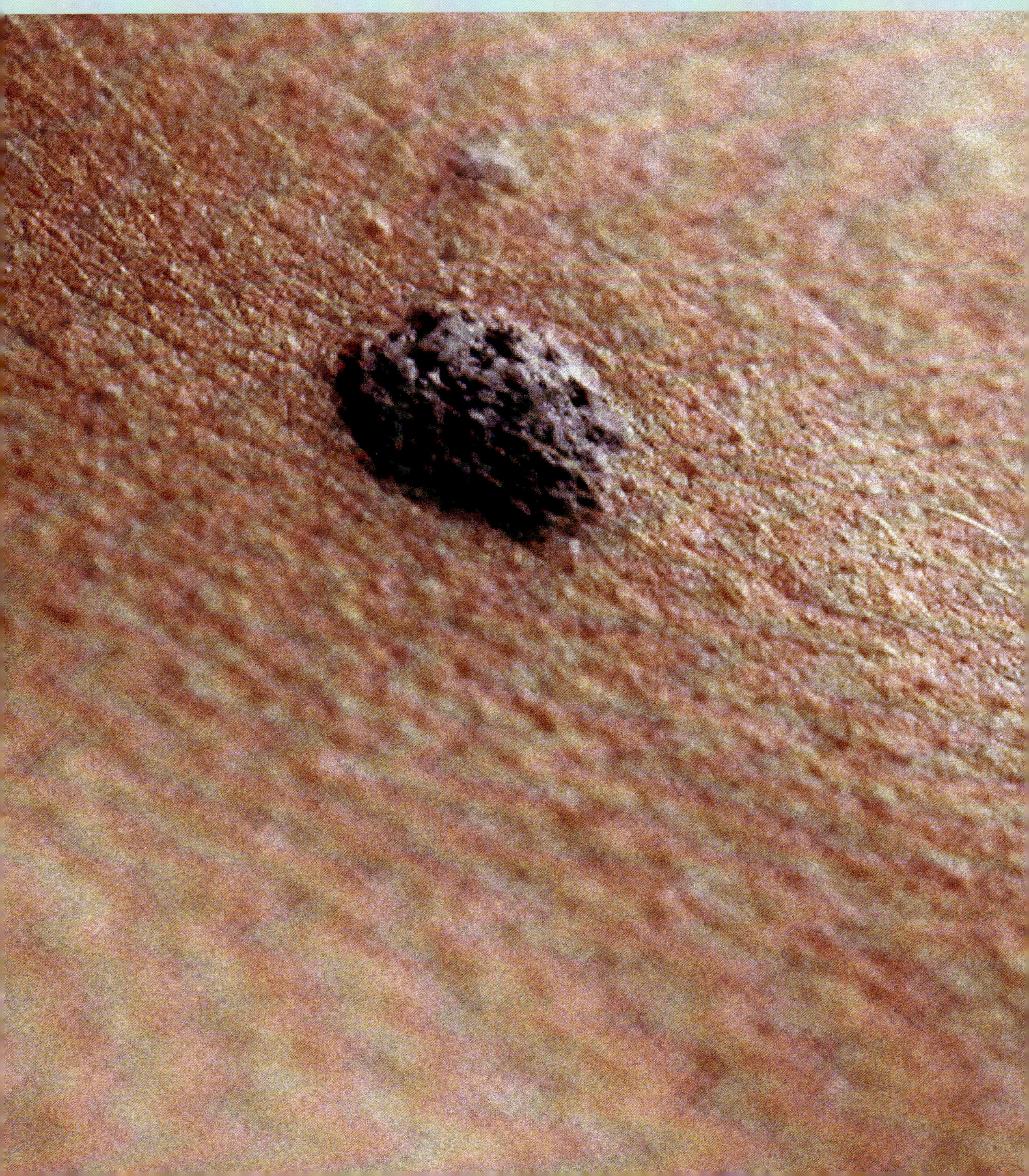

An Overview of Non-melanoma Skin Cancer

Jeffrey P. Larson and Ken R. Wells

In the following selection Jeffrey P. Larson and Ken R. Wells provide an overview of skin cancer, covering aspects such as causes and symptoms for differing types of carcinomas, diagnosis, standard and alternative treatment options, and prognosis. Skin cancer includes several different types of carcinomas, including basal cell, most frequently affecting the face; squamous cell, most common in individuals over forty, and malignant melanoma. According to the authors, cumulative sun exposure is one of the most significant causes of all skin cancers. Standard treatment procedures are used in most non-melanoma cancer cases, while alternative treatments are used more as preventative measures. Larson is a medical writer and registered physical therapist. Wells is a science and business writer.

Photo on previous page. Melanoma usually shows up as a dark-pigmented tumor on the skin. (BSIP/Photo Researchers, Inc.)

Non-melanoma skin cancer is a malignant growth of the external surface or epithelial layer of the skin.

SOURCE: Jeffrey P. Larson and Ken R. Wells, "Skin Cancer, Non-melanoma," *The Gale Encyclopedia of Medicine.* Detroit: 2007. Reproduced by permission of Gale, a part of Cengage Learning.

Skin cancer is the growth of abnormal cells capable of invading and destroying other associated skin cells. Skin cancer is often subdivided into either melanoma or non-melanoma. Melanoma is a dark-pigmented, usually malignant tumor arising from a skin cell capable of making the pigment melanin (a melanocyte). Non-melanoma skin cancer most often originates from the external skin surface as a squamous cell carcinoma or a basal cell carcinoma.

The cells of a cancerous growth originate from a single cell that reproduces uncontrollably, resulting in the formation of a tumor. Exposure to sunlight is documented as the main cause of more than 1 million cases of non-melanoma skin cancer diagnosed each year in the United States. The incidence increases for those living where direct sunshine is plentiful, such as near the equator.

Basal cell carcinoma affects the skin's basal layer and has the potential to grow progressively larger in size, although it rarely spreads to distant areas (metastasizes). Basal cell carcinoma accounts for 80% of skin cancers (excluding melanoma), whereas squamous cell cancer makes up about 20%. Squamous cell carcinoma is a malignant growth of the external surface of the skin. Squamous cell cancers metastasize at a rate of 2–6%, with up to 10% of lesions affecting the ear and lip.

Causes and Symptoms

Cumulative sun exposure is considered a significant risk factor for non-melanoma skin cancer. There is evidence suggesting that early, intense exposure causing blistering sunburn in childhood may also play an important role in the cause of non-melanoma skin cancer. Basal cell carcinoma most frequently affects the skin of the face, with the next most common sites being the ears, the backs of the hands, the shoulders, and the arms. It is prevalent in both sexes and most commonly occurs in people over 40.

About 1–2% of all skin cancers develop within burn scars; squamous cell carcinomas account for about 95% of these cancers, with 3% being basal cell carcinomas and the remainder malignant melanomas.

Basal cell carcinomas usually appear as small skin lesions that persist for at least three weeks. This form of non-melanomatous skin cancer looks flat and waxy, with the edges of the lesion translucent and rounded. The edges also contain small fresh blood vessels. An ulcer in the center of the lesion gives it a dimpled appearance. Basal cell carcinoma lesions vary from 4–6mm in size, but can slowly grow larger if untreated.

Squamous cell carcinoma also involves skin exposed to the sun, such as the face, ears, hands, or arms. This form of non-melanoma is also most common among people over 40. Squamous cell carcinoma presents itself as a small, scaling, raised bump on the skin with a crusting ulcer in the center, but without pain and itching.

Basal cell and squamous cell carcinomas can grow more easily when people have a suppressed immune system because they are taking immunosuppressive drugs or are exposed to radiation. Some people must take immunosuppressive drugs to prevent the rejection of a

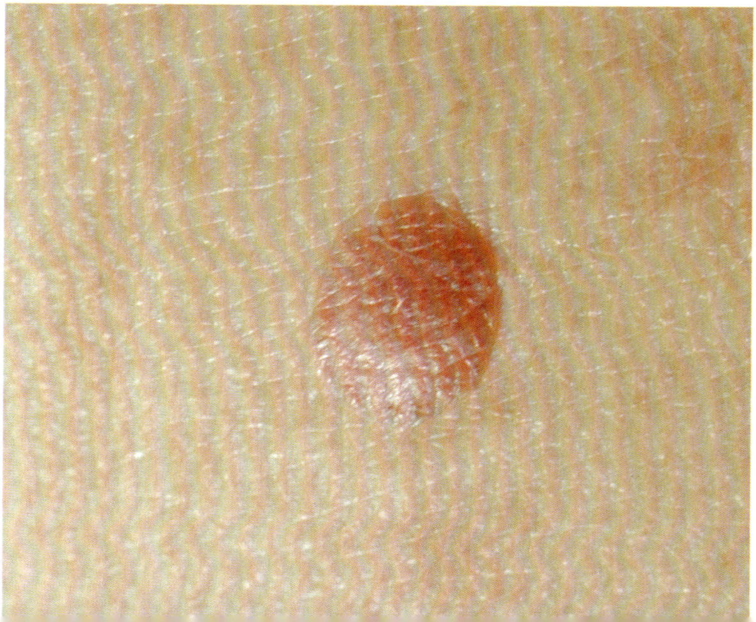

Non-melanoma skin cancer in the form of basal cell carcinoma usually appears as a small skin lesion. (**Chris Bjornberg/Photo Researchers, Inc.**)

transplanted organ or because they have a disease in which the immune system attacks the body's own tissues (autoimmune illnesses); others may need radiation therapy to treat another form of cancer. Because of this, everyone taking these immunosuppressive drugs or receiving radiation treatments should undergo complete skin examination at regular intervals. If proper treatment is delayed and the tumor continues to grow, the tumor cells can spread (metastasize) to muscle, bone, nerves, and possibly the brain.

Diagnosis of Skin Cancer

To diagnose skin cancer, doctors must carefully examine the lesion and ask the patient about how long it has been there, whether it itches or bleeds, and other questions about the patient's medical history. If skin cancer cannot be ruled out, a sample of the tissue is removed and examined under a microscope (a biopsy). A definitive diagnosis of squamous or basal cell cancer can only be made with microscopic examination of the tumor cells. Once skin cancer has been diagnosed, the stage of the disease's development is determined. The information from the biopsy and staging allows the physician and patient to plan for treatment and possible surgical intervention.

FAST FACT

According to the Skin Cancer Foundation, about 1 million cases of basal cell carcinoma are diagnosed annually.

Treatment Options Available Now

A variety of treatment options are available for those diagnosed with non-melanoma skin cancer. Some carcinomas can be removed by cryosurgery, the process of freezing with liquid nitrogen. Uncomplicated and previously untreated basal cell carcinoma of the trunk and arms is often treated with curettage and electrodesiccation, which is the scraping of the lesion and the destruction of any remaining malignant cells with an electrical current. Removal of a lesion

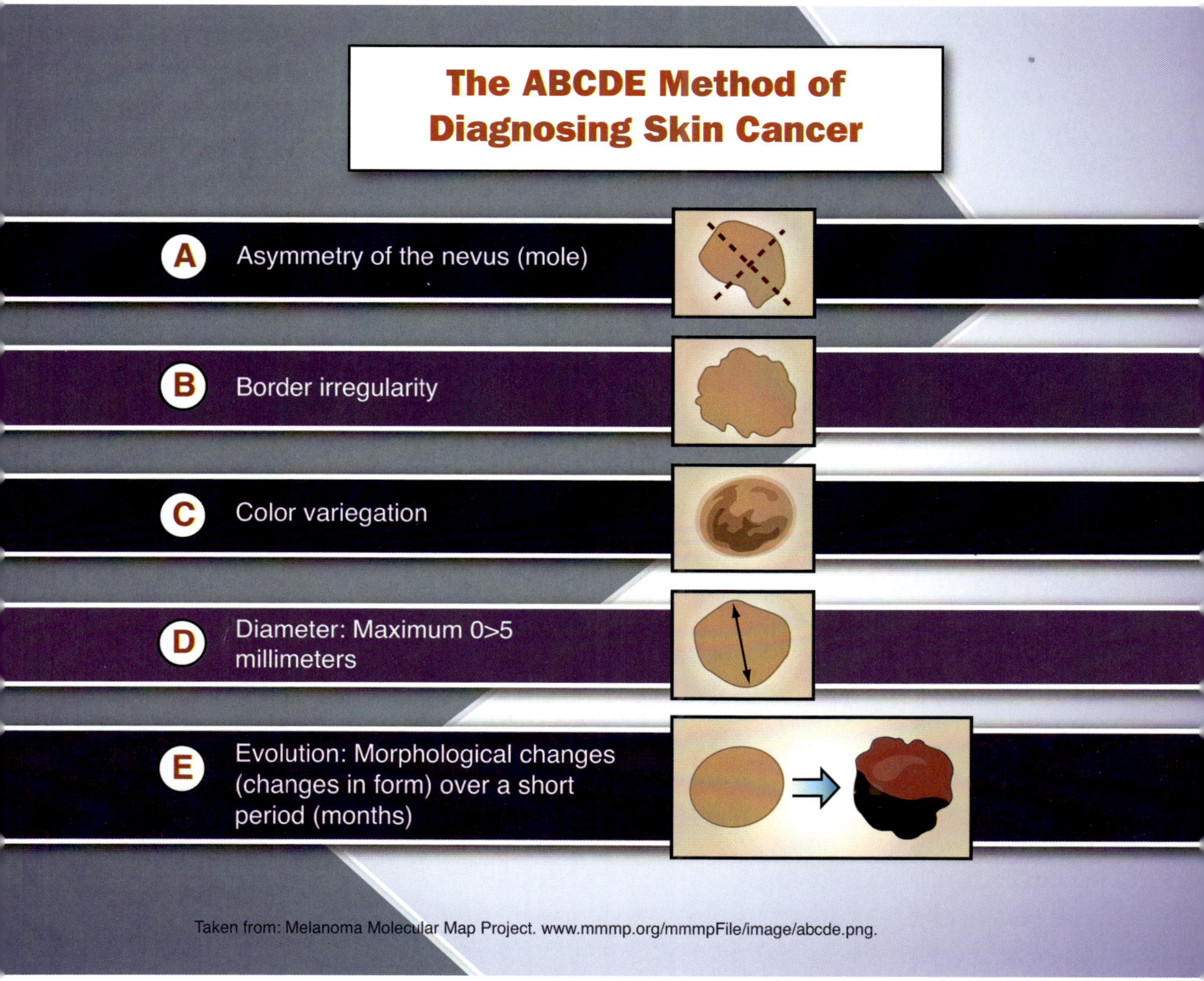

Taken from: Melanoma Molecular Map Project. www.mmmp.org/mmmpFile/image/abcde.png.

layer-by-layer down to normal margins (Mohs' surgery) is an effective treatment for both basal and squamous cell carcinoma. Radiation therapy is best reserved for older, debilitated patients or when the tumor is considered inoperable. Laser therapy is sometimes useful in specific cases; however, this form of treatment is not widely used to treat skin cancer.

A newer type of radiation treatment for non-melanoma skin cancers consists of low-energy x rays delivered through the tip of a portable needle-like probe at a high dosage rate. This method allows the radiologist to treat the cancer while sparing the surrounding normal skin. The device was effective in treating 83% of skin lesions in a group of patients diagnosed with non-melanomatous skin cancers during a Phase I trial for the Food and Drug Administration (FDA). There were no cases of damage to surrounding tissues.

Some topical (applied onto the skin) creams and ointments may be used to treat certain types of non-melanoma skin cancers. For example, imiquimod cream, a topical immune stimulator, has been shown effective in treating superficial basal cell carcinoma. . . .

Alternative Treatment Options, Including Antioxidants

Alternative medicine aims to prevent rather than treat skin cancer. Vitamins have been shown to prevent sunburn and, possibly, skin cancer. Some dermatologists have suggested that taking vitamins E and C may help prevent sunburn. In one particular study, men and women took these vitamins for eight days prior to being exposed to ultraviolet light. The researchers found that those who consumed vitamins required about 20% more ultraviolet light to induce sunburn than did people who didn't take vitamins. This is the first study that indicates the oral use of vitamins E and C increases resistance to sunburn. These antioxidants are thought to reduce the risk of skin cancer, and are expected to provide protection from the sun even in lower doses. Other antixidant nutrients, including beta carotene, selenium, zinc, and the bioflavonoid quercetin have been suggested as possibly preventing skin cancer. However, a 2003 study reported that selenium was not effective in preventing basal cell carcinoma and may even increase risk of squamous cell carcinoma and total non-melanoma skin cancer. Antioxidant herbs such as bilberry (*Vaccinium myrtillus*), hawthorn (*Crataegus laevigata*), tumeric (*Curcuma longa*), and ginkgo (*Ginkgo biloba*) also have been presented as helpful in preventing skin cancers.

A team of researchers at Duke University reported in 2003 that topical application of a combination of 15% vitamin C and 1% vitamin E over a four-day period offered significant protection against sunburn. The researchers suggest that this combination may protect skin against aging caused by sunlight as well.

Another antioxidant that appears to counter the effects of severe sun exposure is superoxide dismutase, or SOD. SOD must be given in injectable form, however, because it is destroyed in the digestive tract.

Researchers are also looking at botanical compounds that could be added to skin care products applied externally to lower the risk of skin cancer. Several botanical compounds [have] been tested on animals and found to be effective in preventing skin cancer, but further research needs to be done on human subjects.

Prognosis and Prevention

Both squamous and basal cell carcinoma are curable with appropriate treatment, although basal cell carcinomas have about a 5% rate of recurrence. Early detection remains critical for a positive prognosis. Although it is rare for basal cell carcinomas to metastasize, their metastases can rapidly lead to death if they invade the eyes, ears, mouth, or the membranes covering the brain.

Avoiding exposure to the sun reduces the incidence of non-melanoma skin cancer. Sunscreen with a sun-protective factor of 15 or higher is helpful in prevention, along with a hat and clothing to shield the skin from sun damage. People should examine their skin monthly for unusual lesions, especially if previous skin cancers have been experienced.

Advances in photographic technique have now made it easier to track the development of moles with the help of whole-body photographs. A growing number of hospitals are offering these photographs as part of outpatient mole-monitoring services.

An Overview of Melanoma

Richard A. McCartney and Ken R. Wells

Malignant melanoma comes from the skin cells that produce melanin. It is the deadliest type of skin cancer and has four distinct subtypes: superficial spreading, nodular, lentigo maligna, and acral lentiginous melanomas, and may appear anywhere on the body. The authors state that most melanoma cases are caused by either environmental factors or genetic predisposition. Suspicious moles can be evaluated with two separate scales; the ABCDE rule or the Glasgow 7-point scale. Each scale takes into account various changes in the look and feel of a mole. The most successful treatments are based on an early diagnosis and can include staging, surgical intervention, tumor management, chemotherapy, and other biological response therapies. Richard A. McCartney is a fellow with the American College of Surgeons, and Ken R. Wells is a science and business writer.

Malignant melanoma is a type of cancer arising from the melanocyte cells of the skin. Melanocytes are cells in the skin that produce a pig-

SOURCE: Richard A. McCartney and Ken R. Wells, *The Gale Encyclopedia of Medicine.* Belmont, CA: Gale, 2007. Reproduced by permission of Gale, a part of Cengage Learning.

ment called melanin. Malignant melanoma develops when the melanocytes no longer respond to normal control mechanisms of cellular growth. They may then invade nearby structures or spread to other organs in the body (metastasis), where again they invade and compromise the function of that organ.

Description

Melanocytes are derived from a structure in the human embryo called the neural crest. They are distributed in the epidermis and thus are found throughout the skin. They produce a brown pigment known as melanin and are responsible for racial variation in skin color as well as the color of moles. Malignant degeneration of the melanocyte

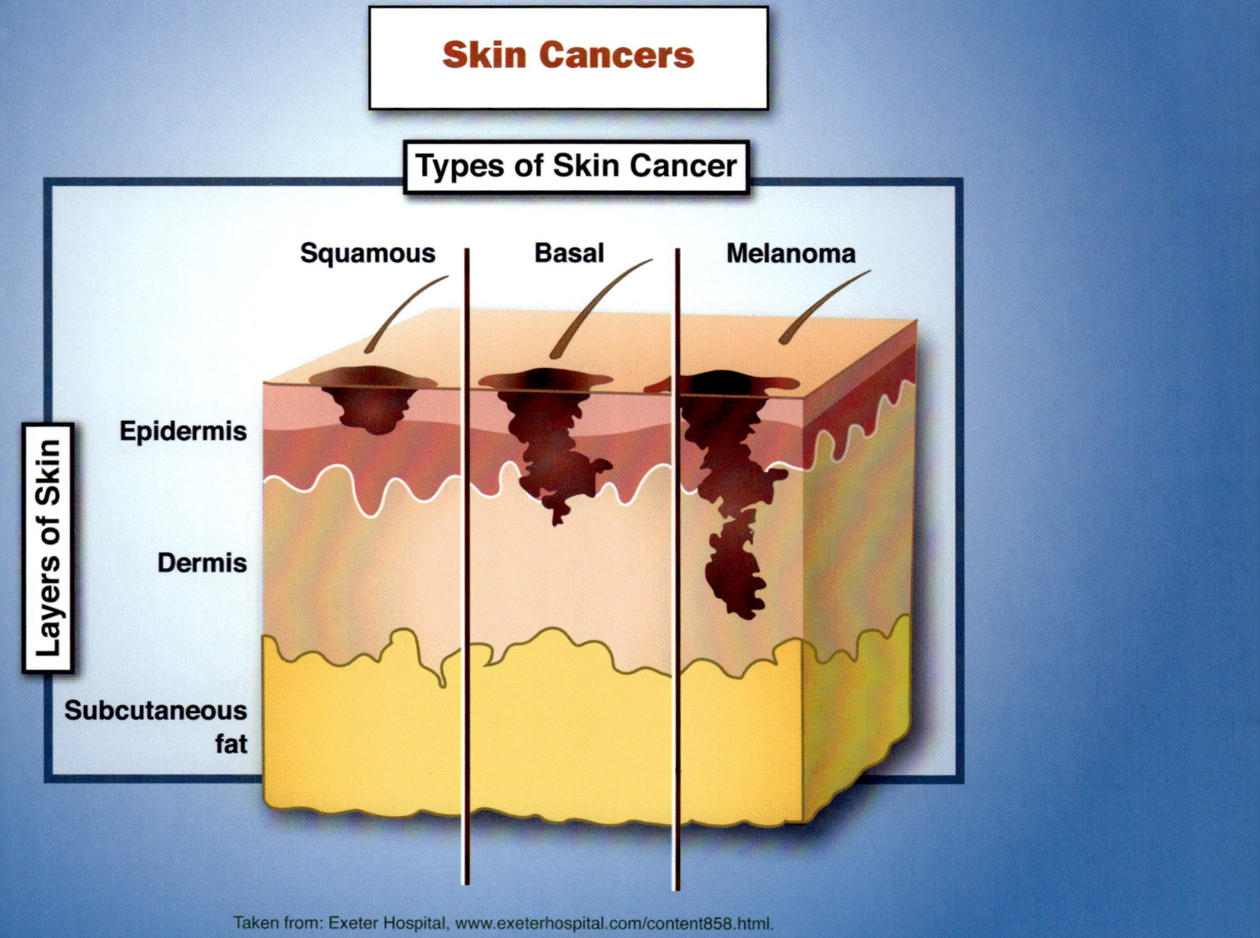

Taken from: Exeter Hospital, www.exeterhospital.com/content858.html.

gives rise to the tumor known as melanoma, which has four subtypes. These are: superficial spreading, nodular, lentigo maligna, and acral lentiginous melanomas, accounting for 70%, 15% to 30%, 4% to 10%, and 2% to 8% of cases, respectively. Malignant melanoma may develop anywhere on the body. In men, it is most common on the trunk. In women, it is most common on the back or legs. The subtype also may influence where the tumor develops; lentigo melanoma is more common on the face while acral lentiginous melanoma is more common on the palms of the hand, soles of the feet, or in the nail beds.

The locally invasive characteristic of this tumor involves vertical penetration through the skin and into the dermis and subcutaneous (under-the-skin) tissues of the malignant melanocytes. With the exception of the nodular variety of melanoma, there is often a phase of radial [from the center outward] or lateral [to the sides] growth associated with these tumors. Since it is the vertical growth that characterizes the malignancy, the nodular variant of melanoma carries the worst prognosis. Fortunately, the superficial spreading type is most common.

Progression of the Tumor

The primary tumor begins in the skin, often from the melanocytes of a pre-existing mole. Once it becomes invasive, it may progress beyond the site of origin to the regional lymph nodes or travel to other organ systems in the body and become systemic in nature.

Lymph is the clear, protein-rich fluid that bathes the cells throughout our body. Lymph will work its way back to the bloodstream via small channels known as lymphatics. Along the way, the lymph is filtered through cellular stations known as nodes, thus they are called lymph nodes. Nearly all organs in the body have a primary lymph node group filtering the tissue fluid, or lymph, that comes from that organ. Different areas of the skin have different primary nodal stations. For the leg, they are in the groin. For the arm, the armpit or axilla. For the face, it is the neck. Depending where on the torso the tumor develops, it may drain into one groin or armpit, or both.

Cancer, as it invades in its place of origin, may also work its way into blood vessels. If this occurs, it provides yet another route for the cancer to spread to other organs of the body. When the cancer spreads elsewhere in the body, it has become systemic in extent and the tumor growing elsewhere is known as a metastasis.

Untreated malignant melanoma follows a classic progression. It begins and grows locally, penetrating vertically.

One of four subtypes of malignant melanoma, nodular melanoma is the most virulent form of skin cancer (**Biophoto Associates/Photo Researchers, Inc.**)

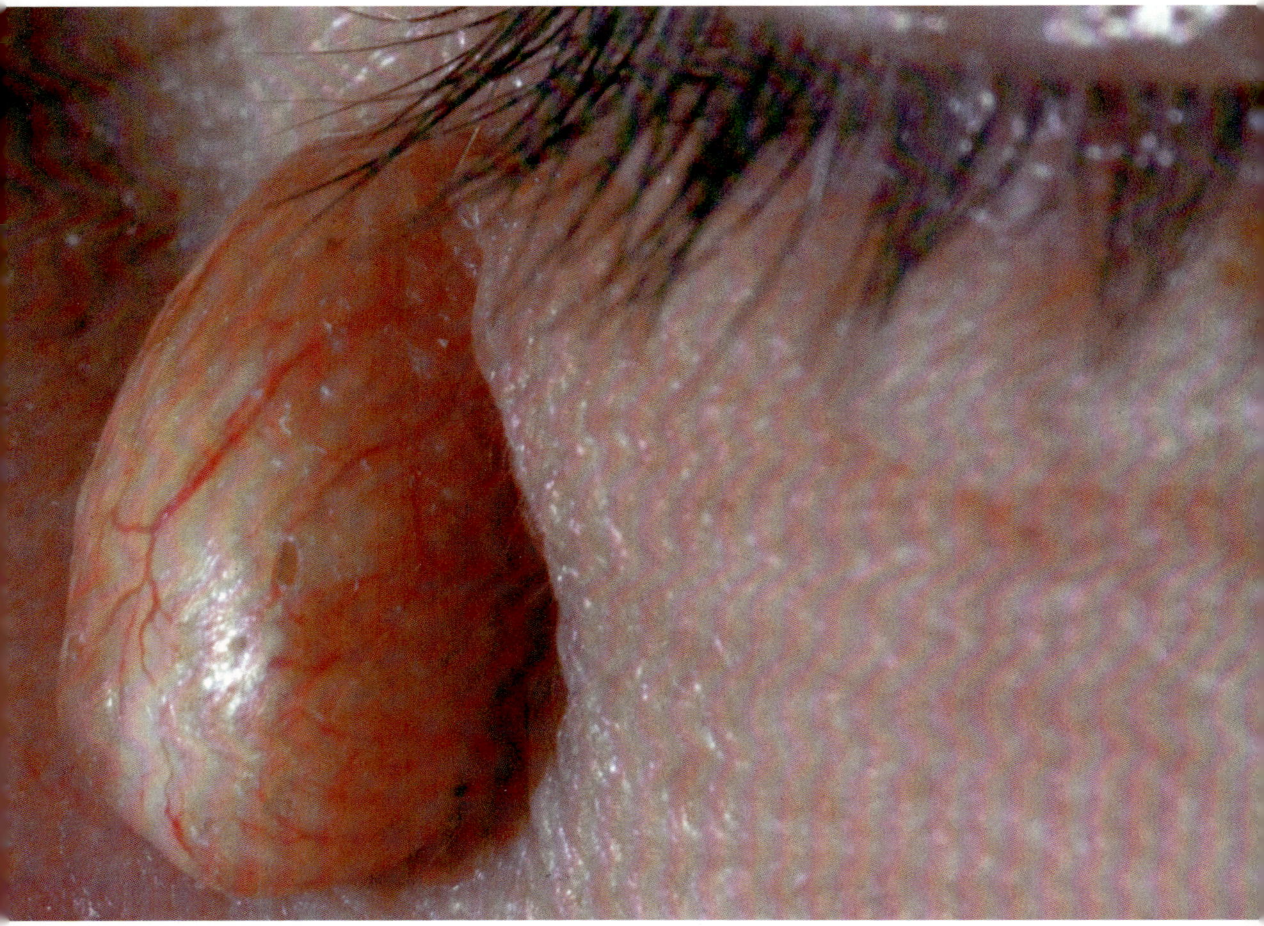

It may be carried via the lymph to the regional nodes, known as regional metastasis. It may go from the lymph to the bloodstream or penetrate blood vessels, directly allowing it a route to go elsewhere in the body. When systemic disease or distant metastasis occur, melanoma commonly involves the lung, brain, liver, or occasionally bone. The malignancy causes death when its uncontrolled growth compromises vital organ function. . . .

The Impact of Sun Exposure

The incidence of primary cutaneous malignant melanoma has been steadily increasing, possibly related to increase of sun exposure. Currently, the risk is about 13 per 100,000 of the population. It affects all age groups but is most commonly seen in patients between 30 and 60 years of age.

Sun exposure definitely increases the risk of developing melanoma, particularly in older males. The melanocytes are part of the integument's [enveloping layer, i.e., skin] photoprotective mechanism; in response to sunlight, they produce melanin that has a protective role from the sun's ultraviolet rays. For Caucasians, the amount of melanin present in the skin is directly related to sun exposure. However, it is not so much the total sun exposure that seems important, rather it is the history of sunburn, (especially if severe or at an early age), that correlates with the increased risk. On this basis populations of fair-skinned people living in areas of high sun exposure such as the southwest United States or Australia are subject to increased risk. Malignant melanoma also affects non-Caucasians—though sun exposure probably does not play a role—at a rate of 10% that of Caucasians. The most common form of melanoma in African Americans is acral lentiginous melanoma.

FAST FACT

According to Harvard University, approximately one out of every twenty people who have had melanoma will develop melanoma again within twenty years.

Malignant melanoma may arise in the skin anywhere on the body. It is estimated that 50%–70% develop spontaneously while the remainder start in a pre-existing mole.

Causes and Symptoms

The predisposing causes to the development of malignant melanoma are environmental and genetic. The environmental factor is excessive sun exposure. There are also genetically transmitted familial syndromes with alterations in the CDKN2A gene, which encodes for the tumor-suppressing proteins p16 and p19. In 2003 a group of Swedish researchers reported that 63 out of a group of 71 melanoma patients, or 89% of the group, had mutations in either the NRAS or the BRAF gene. The researchers found that these mutations occur at an early point in the development of melanoma and remain as the tumor progresses.

As of early 2003, some researchers think there may be two pathways to malignant melanoma, one involving exposure to sunlight and the other with melanocyte proliferation triggered by other factors. This hypothesis is based on the difference in distribution of moles on the body between patients who develop melanomas on the face and neck, and those who develop melanomas on the trunk.

A small percentage of melanomas arise within burn scar tissue. As of 2003, researchers do not fully understand the relationship between deep burns and an increased risk of skin cancer.

As mentioned previously, melanin production in fair-skinned people is induced by sun exposure. An exposure substantial enough to result in mild sunburn will be followed by melanin producing a tan that may last a few weeks. Both ultraviolet radiation and damaging oxygen radicals caused by sun exposure may damage cells, particularly their DNA. It is suspected that this damage induces mutations that result in the development of malignant melanoma. Though these mutations are alterations of the genome causing the melanoma, they are environmentally induced and account for sporadic or spontaneous cases of this disease.

A positive family history of one or two first-degree relatives having had melanoma substantially increases the risk on a genetic basis. A family tendency is observed in 8% to 12% of patients. There is a syndrome known as the dysplastic (atypical) nevus syndrome that is characterized by atypical moles with bothersome clinical features in children under age 10. Such individuals have to be observed closely for the development of malignant melanoma. Chromosome 9p has been identified as being involved in familial predisposition. There are mutations in up to 50% of familial melanoma patients of the tumor-suppressing gene CDKN2A. The actual number of moles increases risk, but the size of the moles needs be considered. Those with 10 larger moles of over 1 cm (0.4 in.) are at more risk than those with a higher number (50–99) of smaller moles. Finally, when a child is born with a large congenital mole, careful observation for change is appropriate because of increased risk.

Rules for Changing Moles

An excellent way of identifying changes of significance in a mole is the ABCDE rule:

- Asymmetry
- Border irregularity
- Color variegation
- Diameter greater than 6 mm (0.24 in)
- Elevation above surrounding tissue.

Notice that three of the criteria refer to variability of the lesion (color variegation refers to areas of light color and black scattered within the mole). Thus small, uniform regular lesions have less cause for concern. It is important to realize that change in a mole or the rapid development of a new one are very important symptoms.

Another summary of important changes in a mole is the Glasgow 7-point scale. The symptoms and signs below can occur anywhere on the skin, including the palms of the hands, soles of the feet, and also the nail beds:

- Change in size
- Change in shape
- Change in color
- Inflammation
- Crusting and bleeding
- Sensory change
- Diameter greater than 7 mm (0.28 in.)

In this scheme, change is emphasized along with size. Bleeding and sensory changes are relatively late symptoms.

Symptoms related to the presence of regional disease are mostly those of nodules or lumps in the areas containing the lymph nodes draining the area. Thus nodularity can be found in the armpit, the groin, or the neck if regional nodes are involved. There is also a special type of metastasis that can occur regionally with malignant melanoma; it is known as an in-transit metastases. If the melanoma is spreading through the lymph system, some of the tumor may grow there, resulting in a nodule part way between the primary site and the original lymph node. These in-transit metastasis are seen both at the time of original presentation or later after primary treatment has been rendered, the latter being a type of recurrence.

Finally, in those who either present with or progress to widespread or systemic disease, symptoms and signs are related to the affected organ. Thus neurological problems, lung problems, or liver problems develop depending on the organ involved.

Diagnosis

None of the clinical signs or symptoms discussed above are absolute indications that a patient has malignant melanoma. The actual diagnosis is accomplished by biopsy, a procedure that removes tissue to examine under a microscope. It is important that the signs and symptoms are used to develop a suspicion of the diagnosis because the way the biopsy is performed for melanoma may be different than for other lesions of the skin.

The doctor may also use a dermatoscope to examine the mole prior to removal. The dermatoscope, which can be used to distinguish between benign moles and melanomas, is an instrument that resembles an ophthalmoscope [for examining the eye]. An immersion oil is first applied to the mole to make the outer layers of skin transparent.

When dealing with an early malignant melanoma, it is very important to establish the exact thickness of penetration of the primary tumor. Any biopsy that does not remove the full vertical extent of the primary is inadequate. Therefore, if a skin lesion is suspicious, full thickness excisional biopsy is the approach recommended. Shave biopsies and biopsies that remove only a portion of the suspect area are inappropriate. Often, in an early case, the excision involves just the suspicious lesion with minimal normal skin, but it should be a full vertical excision of the skin. If a melanoma is diagnosed, further treatment of this area will often be necessary but does not compromise outcome (prognosis). In some special areas of the body, minor modifications may be necessary about initial total excision, but full thickness excision should always be the goal.

Once the diagnosis is obtained, careful examination of the patient for regional lymph node involvement should be done. A careful review to uncover any symptoms of widespread disease is also appropriate.

The more common patient has an early melanoma, and extensive testing is not usually warranted. Routine testing in this situation involves a complete blood count, a chest x ray, and determinations of blood enzymes including lactic dehydrogenase and alkaline phosphatase.

If the patient has signs or symptoms of more advanced disease, or if the lesion's depth of penetration is sizeable, further imaging studies may be appropriate. These would involve CAT [computerized axial tomography]scans of the abdomen, the chest, or regional nodal areas, or a CAT or MRI [magnetic resonance imaging] of the brain.

Treatment and Clinical Staging

The key to successful treatment is early diagnosis. Patients identified with localized, thin, small lesions . . . nearly always survive. For those with advanced lesions, the outcome is poor in spite of progress in systemic therapy.

Malignant melanoma is locally staged based on the depth of penetration through the skin and its appendages. There are two ways of looking at the depth of penetration. The Clarke system utilizes the layers of the dermis and the skin appendages present at that layer to identify the depth of penetration. The Breslow system uses the absolute measurement of depth. Though useful conceptually, the Clarke system is used less frequently because of the fact that skin is of different thickness in different regions of the body. The depth of penetration is much greater when the tumor reaches the subcutaneous fat when the skin involved is the back as opposed to the face. It turns out that the Breslow measurement is more reproducible and thus more useful; therefore, for purposes here, depth of penetration by absolute measurement (Breslow) is used in local staging.

Stage I and stage II have no involvement of the regional lymph nodes and are thus localized to the site of origin. These stages are subdivided on the basis of penetration. Stage Ia is 0.75 mm or less (1 mm=0.04 in), and Stage Ib is 0.75–1.5 mm penetration. Stage IIa is 1.5–4.0 mm and Stage IIb is over 4.0 mm or into the subcutaneous fat. In stage III and IV, there is disease beyond the primary site. Stage III is defined by the presence of in-transit or regional nodal metastasis or both. Stage IV is defined by the presence of distant metastasis.

Once the diagnosis of malignant melanoma has been established by biopsy and the stage has been identified using the results of the examination and studies, a treatment plan is developed. Melanoma is not cured unless it is diagnosed at a stage when it can be isolated and removed surgically. Considerations revolve around the extent of the local and regional nodal surgery for stages I through III. For stage IV patients, or those that are treated and then develop recurrence at distant sites, chemotherapy or immunotherapy is planned. Studies are in progress to improve the results from traditional chemotherapeutic regimens. Adjuvant therapy (auxiliary drug treatment used to make possibility of relapse less for those at high risk) is also considered.

Surgical therapy for the primary site is that of wide local removal of the skin including subcutaneous tissue surrounding the lesion. In the past, wide excisions were large and encompassed 2 in. of tissue in all directions wherever feasible. It has been shown that such wide local excisions are not necessary and the issue has become: how wide is enough? Studies from the World Health Organization Melanoma Group and by the Melanoma Intergroup Committee in the United States have provided general guidelines based on the depth of penetration of the melanoma. These guidelines and anatomic considerations need to be kept in mind by the surgeon.

The Issue of Lymph Nodes

The next issue in primary management is whether the patient should have the regional lymph nodes removed in addition to treatment of the primary tumor. The problems associated with the resection of regional lymph nodes are those of lifelong edema or swelling in the extremity. Though it does not occur in all patients (5% to 20%, depending on the extremity and extent of the dissection), it can be a disabling symptom. Certainly, if it could be ascertained that there was disease in the nodes, resection (removal) would be appropriate. However, if there was no disease, the risk of edema should be avoided. In patients with no signs of regional disease, depth of penetration of the primary tumor helps guide the decision. If the tumor penetrates less than 1 mm, dissection is not usually done. If it is 1–2 mm, node dissection may be done at the time of primary treatment or the patient may be observed and only undergo lymph node dissection if the area later shows signs of disease. If the patient has enlarged lymph nodes or the depth of the tumor has led to the evaluation by CAT scan showing enlarged nodes, resection of the nodes will be considered. In the latter case, more extensive imaging of the lung, liver, or brain may be appropriate to be sure the patient does not already have stage IV disease.

Questions related to which patients should have resection of regional lymph nodes have led to an intermediary procedure known as sentinel node mapping and biopsy. Intermediate thickness melanomas between 1 and 4 mm deep (0.04 and 0.16 in.) may have nodal involvement even if the examination and any other studies done are normal. If a radioisotope tracer or blue dye is injected into the area of the primary tumor, very shortly it will travel to the lymph nodes draining that area. These sentinel nodes are thus identifiable and are the most likely to harbor any regional metastatic disease. If these nodes alone are biopsied and are normal, the rest of the lymph node group can be spared. If they show microscopic deposits of tumor, then the full resection of the lymph node group may be completed. This procedure allows selection of those patients with intermediate thickness melanoma who will benefit from the regional lymph node dissection.

Other Treatments

Patients with metastatic melanoma who do not respond well to other therapies may be candidates for treatment with aldesleukin. Aldesleukin is a form of interleukin, a specific kind of biological response modifier that promotes the development of T-cells. These cells are part of the lymphatic system and can directly interact with and fight cancer cells. Although aldesleukin is produced naturally in the body, its therapeutic form is developed via biotechnology in a laboratory setting. Treatment is considered palliative, which means that it provides comfort but does not produce a cure. Side effects, however, can be severe, and range from flu-like symptoms to whole-body infection (sepsis) and coma.

Some patients, such as those with [stage] II or stage III melanoma, are at high risk for the development of recurrence after treatment. Although these patients are clinically free of disease after undergoing primary treatment, they are more likely to have some microscopic disease in the body that studies have not yet been able to identify. In an effort to decrease the rate of relapse, adjuvant therapy may be considered. Interferon alpha 2a is an agent that stimulates the immune system. This adjuvant therapy may slightly increase the duration of a patient's disease-free state and lengthen overall survival. However, interferon alpha 2a has high toxicity and patients may not tolerate the side effects.

Unfortunately, treatment for those patients who present with or go on to develop systemic disease usually fails; **melanoma** that has metastasized to the brain is particularly difficult to treat. The chemotherapeutic agent dacarbazine, or DTIC, seems to be the most active agent. Overall responses are noted in about 20% of patients, and they last only two to six months. Combination therapy may be an option. The regimen of DTIC+BCNU (carmustine)+cisplatin+tamoxifen delivers a response rate of 40%. Combining biologic or immunologic agents such as interferon with standard chemotherapeutic agents is under study and showing improved response rates, though toxicity is substantial and only the healthier, younger patients tolerate the treatment.

Some researchers are investigating the reasons why melanomas are so resistant to chemotherapy. One suggestion is that the genes ordinarily responsible for apoptosis (cell self-destruction) do not function normally in melanomas. The development of new drugs to treat melanoma depends on a better understanding of the complex processes involved in apoptosis. As of 2007, several new drugs were in development. The most promising seemed to be Zadazin (thymalfasin) when used in combination with standard dacarbazine (DTIC) chemotherapy.

Though radiation therapy has a minimal role in the primary treatment of malignant melanoma, for patients who have metastatic disease, radiation may be helpful. This is true in patients who have developed tumor deposits in such areas as the brain or bone.

Prognosis and Prevention

Almost all patients survive stage Ia malignant melanoma, and the survivorship for stage I overall is more than 90%. Survival drops in stage IIa to about 65% at five years and is worse yet for stage IIb at slightly over 50%. Stage III has a survival rate at 5 years of 10%–47%, depending on the size and number of regional nodes involved. Stage IV malignant melanoma is almost always a fatal disease.

For those with familial tendencies for malignant melanoma, genetic counseling may be appropriate. Psychological counseling may be appropriate for anyone having trouble coping with a potentially fatal disease. Local cancer support groups may be helpful and are often identified by contacting local hospitals or the American Cancer Society.

Though it is difficult to prove that sunscreens statistically reduce the frequency of malignant melanoma at this time, most authorities recommend their use as protection from ultraviolet light (considered a major factor in the development of melanoma.) Avoidance of severe sunburns is recommended.

The Risk Factors for Melanoma

Jill R. Schofield and William A. Robinson

In the following selection the various and multiple risk factors for melanoma are discussed in detail. Authors Jill R. Schofield and William A. Robinson explain that differing moles are normally what lead to melanoma, including number of moles, changing moles, and atypical moles. Other risk factors include prior severe sunburns, sun exposure, family members with melanoma, skin type, age, and other health issues. According to the authors, one of the greatest risk factors is having atypical mole syndrome, which is characterized by having a minimum of one hundred moles on the body with at least ten of them being atypical. Schofield is an internist at St. Joseph Hospital in Denver, Colorado. Robinson is a professor of clinical oncology at the University of Colorado.

We know that melanoma is associated with sun exposure, but we also know that some people are more likely than others to develop melanoma, even when they have the same amount of ex-

SOURCE: Jill R. Schofield and William A. Robinson, *What You Really Need to Know About Moles and Melanoma.* Baltimore: The Johns Hopkins University Press, 2000.

posure to the sun. By comparing large groups of people who have or have not contracted melanoma, physicians have discovered a number of personal characteristics that are associated with it. These characteristics are known as risk factors. Being familiar with these risk factors is extremely important.

People at high risk for melanoma need to be especially careful to implement preventive measures. They and their doctors must also be vigilant in looking for changes that may signal the onset of melanoma, so that any occurrence of the disease can be detected as early as possible. . . . We will discuss the most important risk factors for the development of melanoma. . . .

Changing Moles and Number of Moles

A mole that is changing in any way is of concern and should always be evaluated by a professional. . . .

The more moles you have, the greater your risk for developing melanoma. This is true even if none of your moles have atypical or precancerous features. This is really not surprising, since most melanomas seem to develop from moles.

The number of moles a person has is determined by a combination of factors, but the two most important are probably genetics and sun exposure. Researchers have found that identical twins (who have identical genes) usually have similar numbers of moles. Fraternal twins or other siblings (who share only some of their genes) are less likely to resemble each other in this respect, just as they are less likely to have the same hair color or eye color.

There is also little doubt that number of moles is related to sun exposure. . . . Moles (and melanomas) are most common on parts of the body that receive the most intense, intermittent sun. Caucasians living in tropical and subtropical climates have more moles than those residing in temperate climates.

There is also some evidence that the immune system plays a role in determining the number of moles a person has. People infected with the AIDS virus, people who have had organ transplants, and people who have been on medications that suppress the immune system tend to have more moles.

Atypical Moles

Atypical [abnormal] moles may serve as precursors to melanoma, and they also serve as a general marker of people at risk for melanoma. As with benign moles, the more you have, the greater your risk. As many as 5–10% of Caucasians will develop at least one atypical mole in their lifetime, but most of these people do not have atypical mole syndrome. So as long as these atypical moles are removed or closely monitored for change, the increase in their risk is not that great. . . .

Intense, Intermittent Sun Exposure

Surprisingly, outdoor workers have not been shown to be at high risk for developing melanoma. By contrast, people with a high educational and socioeconomic status who have indoor occupations have been. In addition, melanoma is most common on body parts most likely to receive intense, intermittent sun—the back in men and the legs in women (each location accounts for 40% of all melanomas in the respective sexes)—rather than the head, neck, hands, and forearms, areas that receive regular sun exposure.

These observations and others have led researchers to conclude that intense, intermittent sun exposure is a bigger risk factor for melanoma than chronic, steady sun exposure. For example, a lawyer who works indoors 12 hours daily, six days per week, sees very little sun all week. But then, to release stress, he goes for a 4-hour bike ride on Sunday from 10 A.M. to 2 P.M.—the peak hours of UV [ultraviolet] exposure. That same lawyer is also likely to have the financial resources to take frequent vacations in the tropics. Doctors and scientists now believe that repeated episodes of intermittent, intense sun exposure are a real risk factor for melanoma and should be avoided, particularly by people with other risk factors. . . .

Prior Severe Sunburns

Sunburn is the ultimate evidence of intense, intermittent sun exposure, and almost every epidemiological study ever done on melanoma has shown that a history of severe sunburns in childhood is associated with an increased risk of melanoma. The more times you have been sunburned, the greater the likelihood that you have set the stage for melanoma to develop. Each sunburn causes major damage to the DNA of the skin cells, and the damage accumulates with each burn, since melanocytes last a lifetime.

The ill effects of sunburn—which include wrinkles, lots of ugly spots, and nonmelanoma skin cancer, in addition

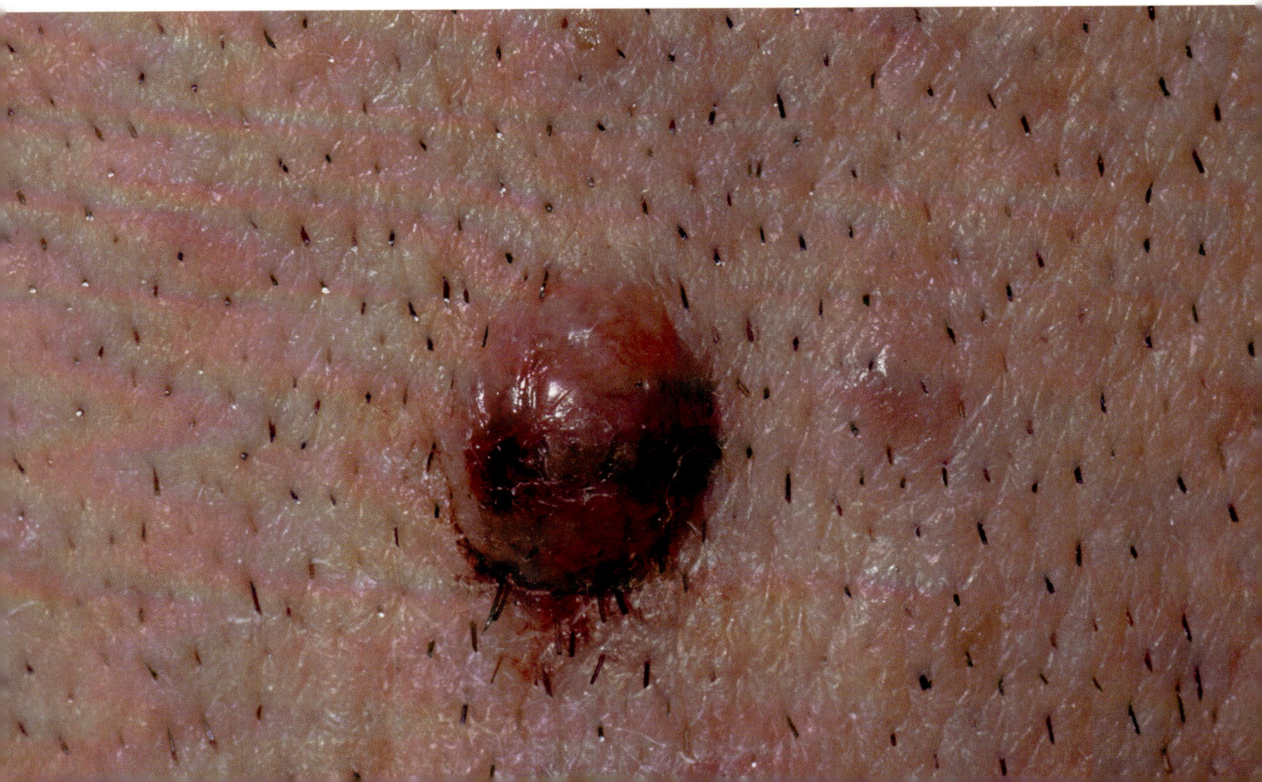

Moles usually develop in childhood or early adulthood. Having large numbers of moles increases a person's risk of developing melanoma. (**Dr. P. Marazzi/Photo Researchers, Inc.**)

to melanoma—usually do not show up for many years. There is therefore no immediate incentive (other than the discomfort of the sunburn) for young people to discontinue their bad sun habits. By the time they are adults, they will probably experience far less sun exposure, but unfortunately the damage has already been done. This is why we urge everyone to teach their children good sun habits early.

Melanoma in a Close Relative

Most people diagnosed with melanoma do not have a family history of the problem. Ten percent of patients, however, do have one or more first-degree relatives with the disease (your first-degree relatives are your parents, your brothers and sisters, and your children). Most of this is not due to a true inheritance of the disease but, rather, to the fact that we often inherit the same skin type and tendency to form moles as our parents; we frequently have had similar amounts of sun exposure as our parents, as well.

By contrast, . . . in rare cases melanoma actually can be inherited. In other words, certain genes that predispose a person to melanoma may be passed on from generation to generation. These inherited gene abnormalities (germline mutations) are relatively uncommon and are usually brought to light when a *number* of family members over several generations suffer from the disease. For most people the risk associated with having a single first-degree relative who has been diagnosed with melanoma ranges from 2 to 12 times the average risk of getting the disease. For people from a "melanoma family," however, the risk is as high as 100%.

Because of the potential risk, you should get to know your family's medical history and should let family members know if you are diagnosed with melanoma so that they can take appropriate preventive measures.

Personal History of Melanoma

People who have had one melanoma are at greater-than-average risk for developing additional primary melanomas. For most melanoma patients this risk is about 1–5%, but for people with the atypical mole syndrome the risk is much higher. All melanoma patients should take extra care in getting to know their remaining moles and examining them regularly. They should also have full skin examinations at regular intervals (at least every 6 months), with removal of any worrisome lesions. Fortunately, most melanoma patients are vigilant and know what signs to look for, so most of these subsequent melanomas are discovered early and removed before they become dangerous.

Skin Type and Hair Color

A common characteristic of melanoma patients is fair skin. Indeed, the likelihood of developing melanoma is directly related to skin color—the lighter your skin, the greater your risk. That being said, however, there are still many Caucasians with skin that tans easily who develop melanoma. Even people with naturally dark skin, such as Africans and Indians, occasionally get the disease, though this is uncommon.

There is a common misconception that most people who develop melanoma have red hair, probably because we often associate redheads with fair skin. Although the percentage of melanoma patients who have red hair (12–15% in the United States) is higher than the percentage of redheads in the general population (6–8%), most melanoma patients in the United States have light to medium brown or blonde hair. The percentage of melanoma patients with red hair may be higher in Australia and Britain due to a greater percentage of redheads in their populations.

Age and Gender

Although much of the skin damage that leads to melanoma occurs early in life, when we receive most of our sun exposure, most melanomas do not appear until adulthood. The risk of developing melanoma, like the risk of most cancers, increases with advancing age. In the past, the average age at the time of diagnosis of melanoma was 45, but recent years have seen a decline in age at diagnosis, with many people now developing melanoma in their 20s and 30s. . . . Melanoma is the most common form of cancer in Australian males aged 25–59 and is second only to breast cancer in females in the same age group. It is also the second most common form of cancer in both males and females aged 15–24. This trend is thought to reflect greater sun exposure earlier in life. Melanoma in children is uncommon but not unheard of. . . .

There is no evidence that one sex is more prone to melanoma than the other. On average, women who do get the disease have slightly fewer recurrences than men. A trend toward increasing incidence in men, particularly in Australia, is probably due to changing lifestyles.

Suppression of the Immune System

We have learned only in the last decade that people with a suppressed or weakened immune system seem to be at an increased risk for developing melanoma. Specifically, people who require immuno-suppressive treatment after a bone marrow or organ transplant and people infected with the AIDS virus have been shown in scientific studies to have an increased likelihood of developing melanoma. Because weakening of the immune system has only recently been identified as a risk factor for melanoma, few details are known. It is curious though, as we have already mentioned, that these same people tend to develop more moles. More studies will certainly be done to investigate this risk factor further.

Prior PUVA Treatments to the Skin

PUVA (an abbreviation for "psoralen and ultraviolet A") is a specialized type of ultraviolet light therapy used to treat severe forms of the skin disorder psoriasis. Not surprisingly, patients who have received prolonged PUVA therapy (more than 250 treatments) have more than five times the average risk of developing melanoma. Most of these melanomas occur 15 or more years after the PUVA treatments began.

Xeroderma Pigmentosa

Xeroderma pigmentosa is an extremely rare condition, but you may have heard about it because it is associated with an extremely high risk of developing both melanoma and nonmelanoma skin cancers. This is because affected persons have a defect in what are called *DNA repair enzymes*. These enzymes are the tools used by cells to repair the everyday damage that occurs to our DNA. Without these very important enzymes, skin cells have no hope against the sun's potent UV rays.

Atypical Mole Syndrome

The strongest risk factor for the development of melanoma is the atypical mole syndrome, which is also known as the dysplastic nevus syndrome. Only a small percentage of the Caucasian population have this condition (less than 1%), but it is important because of its close association with melanoma. The syndrome was first described by Dr. Wallace Clark . . . and his colleagues in 1978. They reported the frequent presence of unusual moles in many members of six families with hereditary melanoma. These moles tended to predominate on the upper torso and arms. They were large, averaging 1 centimeter (about half an inch) in diameter, and irregular in outline. Their pigmentation had a very haphazard mixture of pink, tan, and various shades of brown, and they frequently could be felt to have a slightly raised component, although they appeared completely flat to the naked eye. . . .

As if this syndrome didn't already have enough names, you may also hear it referred to as the FAMM syndrome, which stands for *familial atypical mole and melanoma syndrome.* This name is misleading, however, since some persons with the syndrome do not have a family history of melanoma or even a family history of atypical or multiple moles. In fact, there are now considered to be two subtypes of the atypical mole syndrome: familial (or hereditary) and sporadic, in which there do not appear to be other family members with either the atypical mole syndrome or melanoma. Scientists believe that sporadic cases represent a new genetic mutation, rather than one that has been passed on from generation to generation.

Moles May Not Fit Typical Descriptions

Since the initial reports of the atypical mole syndrome, it has become clear that not all people with the syndrome have moles that fit the original . . . mole description. For example, the nevi [chronic lesions of the skin commonly called birth marks or moles] may be smaller and they may not have the striking variability from mole to mole mentioned in the initial report. There may also be an "inverse pattern," particularly in women, where the majority of nevi may be on the legs rather than on the back, chest, and arm. . . . Finally, both the total number of moles and the number of atypical moles can vary significantly from person to person. The wide variability in the nevi observed in people with the atypical mole syndrome is probably due to different genetic mutations. This has not been proved, but it has recently been shown that only 15 % of persons with a history of multiple primary melanomas (many of whom have the atypical mole syn-

Percentage Distribution of Malignant Melanoma on Parts of the Body, by Sex

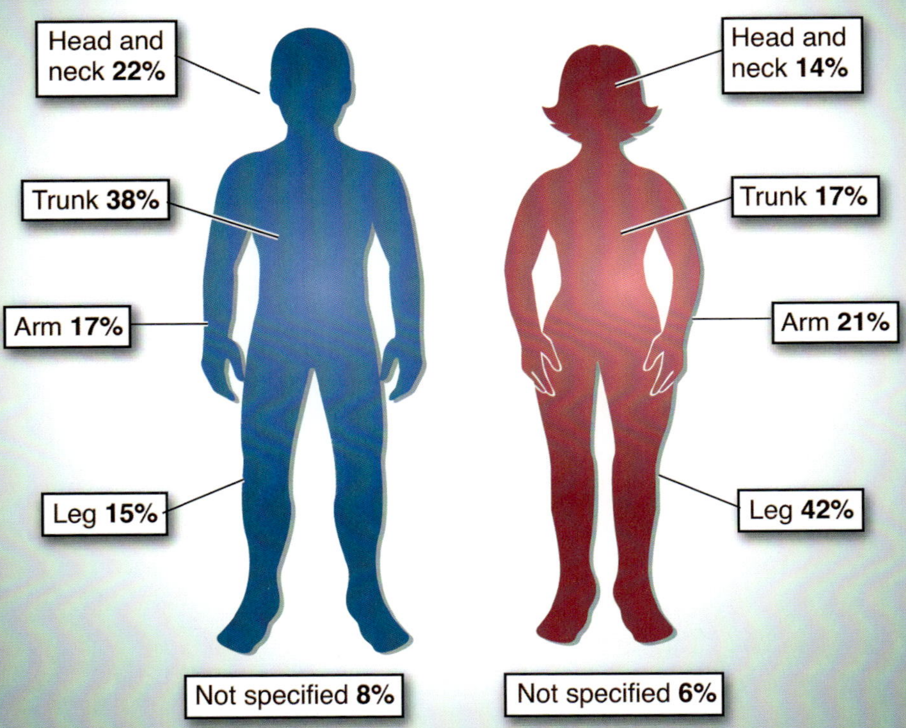

Taken from: Cancer Research United Kingdom.

drome) have inherited an abnormal p16 gene. The assumption is that the other 85 % have different genetic mutations that have not yet been identified, and that each different mutation may express itself in its own distinct way.

Because of the variability of the atypical mole syndrome, it is sometimes difficult to decide whether a patient has the syndrome or not. The most widely accepted criterion is the presence of more than 100 total body moles, at least 10 of which have atypical features when viewed on the skin and/or when examined under a microscope. As you might imagine, the diagnosis is not an exact science. It is difficult to make a precise count of the total number of moles you have or the number with atypical features, especially if you have lots of moles. The experience of the doctor and factors such as a personal or family history of melanoma or atypical nevi play an important role in making a diagnosis. . . .

People who have more than 50 total body moles but do not meet the criteria for the atypical mole syndrome are said to have an abnormal mole pattern. Although they do not have the atypical mole syndrome, these people still have a high risk of developing melanoma. It seems that whatever genetic abnormality results in the propensity to form an unusually large number of nevi also results in a propensity to form mutations leading to atypical or premalignant moles, so the two frequently go hand in hand.

Although . . . *most* people do not acquire new moles after the age of 30, people with the atypical mole syndrome or an abnormal mole pattern frequently continue to acquire new moles throughout adult life, even into their 60s and 70s. In addition, they commonly develop moles in places that are rarely, if ever, exposed to the sun: on the scalp, the feet, the buttocks, the groin, and the female breast. The presence in children of moles in these unusual locations, particularly on the scalp, may be the first indication of the atypical mole syndrome. Removal of nevi on the scalp, even if they do not have worrisome features, may be recommended, since they are difficult to monitor for change. Melanomas that arise on the scalp are frequently very deeply invading at the time of diagnosis because they are not readily noticed at an earlier stage. . . .

Three Risk Groups

What is your risk of developing melanoma if you have atypical moles? The risk ranges widely from as low as 7 times normal to as high as 500 times normal. . . .

There are three different risk groups within this broad range. The lowest risk group includes those who have one or more atypical moles but do not meet the criteria for the atypical mole syndrome. This means people with fewer than 100 total body moles and fewer than ten with atypical features. (Within this subgroup, those with the fewest total moles and the fewest atypical moles are at the lowest risk of all.) The middle risk group includes those who do meet the criteria for the atypical mole syndrome but who have never been diagnosed with melanoma and do not have any close relatives with melanoma. People at highest risk for the development of melanoma are those with the atypical mole syndrome who either have a personal history of one or more prior melanomas and/or have one or more close relatives with melanoma. In fact, it has been estimated that people with the atypical mole syndrome who come from "melanoma kindreds" . . . or who have at least two close relatives with melanoma, have a 100% chance of developing melanoma themselves by the time they reach age 70 unless they are extremely vigilant, take proper sun precautions, and have suspicious lesions removed immediately. In addition, people with the atypical mole syndrome tend to develop melanoma at young ages (the 20s is not uncommon); if not monitored close1y, these people frequently develop multiple invasive melanoma.

FAST FACT

The National Institutes of Health reports that changes caused by ultraviolet radiation in the p53 tumor-suppressing gene have been linked to higher frequencies of skin cancer.

The Treatment of Melanoma

Howard L. Kaufman

One of the main forms of treatment for melanoma is surgery. In the following selection author Howard L. Kaufman describes and explains the processes and conditions that accompany excise surgery, including general descriptive guidelines, how the melanoma is situated, and what kind of surgeons may be involved. In place of excise surgery, other options include laser therapy, cryotherapy, radiation, and topical treatments. According to the author, these other treatments are not the first choice and are often problematic for varying reasons. Kaufman is the founder of the Columbia University Melanoma Center and is the chief of surgical oncology and an associate professor of surgery at Columbia University College of Physicians and Surgeons.

The treatment of primary melanoma (Stage I and II) is surgical excision or removal of all melanoma cells in order to halt its spread. Without treatment, the natural course for melanoma is to grow into deeper layers from its most common primary site, the skin. Once it reaches the mid- to lower dermis, melanoma cells can

SOURCE: Howard L. Kaufman, *The Melanoma Book: A Complete Guide to Prevention and Treatment.* New York: Gotham, 2005.

enter the lymphatic vessels and spread to the local lymph nodes. From the lymph nodes melanoma can then spread to virtually any other organ in the body. In cases where complete removal is possible and no spread has occurred, melanoma can be cured.

Wide Local Excision

The surgical treatment is a wide local excision, in which the entire melanoma and surrounding skin are removed. Exactly how wide is "wide"? The answer depends on how deep into the skin the melanoma has grown. This is an important point; it is not how large the melanoma grows across the surface of the skin but how deep it goes into the dermis that determines the extent of surgery. Therefore, a melanoma relatively large in circumference on the surface of the skin may require less treatment than a tiny nodule that has grown deep into the underlying dermis below the surface of the skin.

The margin, or amount of surrounding skin to be removed as part of a wide local excision, has been the subject of much debate for many years. A large number of clinical studies have compared different margins of skin removal to determine the chances of melanoma returning as well as the chances of living a normal life after the operation. The good news is that over time we have learned that for most melanoma lesions a smaller margin may lead to an equally positive prognosis as a wider margin. The general guidelines that I use are as follows:

- Early melanomas that have not gone deeper than the epidermis, also called in-situ melanoma: a margin of 0.5 centimeters, or about a quarter of an inch.
- Melanomas less than one millimeter deep: a margin of one centimeter, or about half an inch.
- Any melanoma deeper than one millimeter: a margin of two centimeters, or about one inch. . . .

Surgical Margins for Melanomas of Different Depths

Melanoma depth	Incision size	Incision measurement
In-situ		0.5 cm
Thin	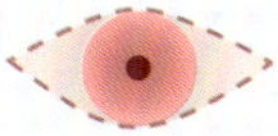	1.0 cm
Thick	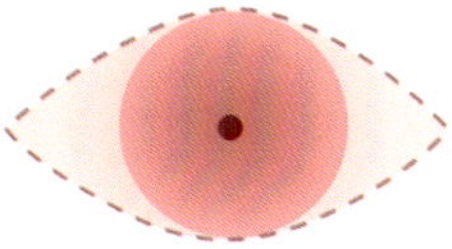	2.0 cm

Taken from: Howard L. Kaufman, *The Melanoma Book*, New York: Gotham, 2005.

The actual incision shape most surgeons use is an ellipse. This shape allows the skin to close back more easily, without the skin having to stretch much. The closure of any surgical incision without tension results in better healing and less scar formation. . . . Sometimes there is some tension or the margins are large enough to cause a major defect. For example, when the primary melanoma is very large in circumference—if a melanoma is four centimeters across and a two centimeter margin is necessary on all sides—the total skin removal will be eight centimeters. While it may still be easy to close if the melanoma is on the back or abdominal wall, it can be difficult if it is on the face or knee cap. In the event that the defect is large we have some tricks that can be used to help bring the skin together, including larger and stronger stitches, a special technique called undermining, or even a skin graft.

Adequate Treatment Is Necessary

An important point: When a melanoma is quite small the entire melanoma may be removed with the biopsy procedure, but *this is not adequate treatment.* It you are suspected of having melanoma, a biopsy is performed to confirm the diagnosis and determine the depth of the melanoma. This information is then used to plan the real treatment procedure—the wide local excision. If you have only had a biopsy, I do not consider the melanoma to have been treated adequately. The biopsy is necessary to determine how deep the melanoma has grown, since this information is used to plan the size of the margins needed as part of the wide local excision.

While many dermatologists are comfortable performing small excisions for melanoma, if the lesion is deep you may need to see a surgical oncologist for treatment. A plastic surgeon might also be needed when complicated closures are required following an excision. It is important to ascertain whether your doctor is familiar with these procedures and whether they perform them frequently. A biopsy is relatively straightforward and simple. Definitive treatment requires a higher level of expertise. . . .

Although wide local excision is the treatment of choice for melanoma, there are other treatment options that may be used in selected cases. . . . Most of these procedures result in the direct destruction of the melanoma within the skin and do not allow a careful pathology review.

Radiation Therapy

Radiation is not commonly used because it does not allow direct examination of the lesion, clear margins cannot be accurately predicted, and the complications are generally more severe than those seen with surgical excision. Nevertheless, there are times when radiation may be very useful as a primary or secondary treatment. Contrary to popular opinion, melanoma cells may be quite sensitive to radiation. Radiation therapy can be used to kill melanoma on the skin and in other sites. I sometimes use radiation for patients with very large melanomas where an operation would result in disfiguring defects. Radiation may also be useful for patients who have a large number of melanoma lesions, which prevents simple excision of the skin. It may take up to two years for melanoma lesions to disappear after radiation treatment. The decision to use radiation should be made on an individual basis and requires discussion between the oncologist, surgeon, and radiation oncologist, who actually performs the procedure.

Laser Therapy

Laser is an acronym that stands for "Light Amplification by Stimulated Emission of Radiation." First developed in the 1960s, laser technology uses either a solid or gas medium that when stimulated induces electromagnetic radiation in the visible light or infrared spectrum. Lasers are used in the medical field to provide a highly focused beam that results in a photothermal effect and vaporizes tissue on contact. The use of laser therapy has little pain and swelling compared to other techniques. Laser therapy has been proposed for the treatment of skin cancers other than melanoma and may be quite useful for small benign tumors. There is little evidence that laser therapy is appropriate for melanoma, however. The major problem with laser therapy is that no tissue is obtained for evaluation and there is no way to confirm that all the melanoma cells have been destroyed. I do not recommend laser therapy for the treatment of primary melanoma except in highly specific circumstances, such as for very small melanomas in patients who cannot have surgery.

Cryotherapy and Mohs Micrographic Surgery

Cryotherapy uses extreme cold to freeze tumor cells and has been useful for some types of cancer. This technique suffers from the same problems as laser therapy and has not been validated for the treatment of melanoma.

Mohs technique was popularized for the treatment of basal cell carcinomas, a more benign skin cancer. Mohs involves the sequential removal of a tumor with immediate microscopic examination to determine if tumor cells are present. The dissection continues as long as the tumor is still present in the specimen. The technique is especially useful for basal cell carcinomas because it allows the complete removal of the tumor without taking any additional skin. This leads to an optimal cosmetic result since the minimum amount of tissue is removed. Mohs technique

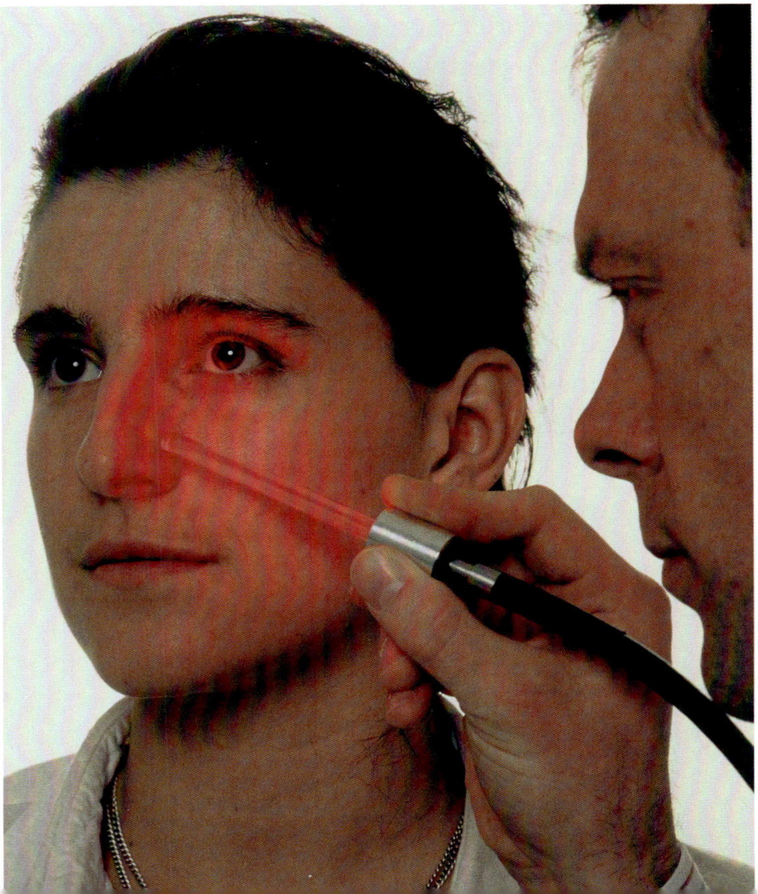

Photodynamic therapy, one of several methods of skin cancer treatment, involves applying a special cancer-killing cream that is activated by light. (David Parker/ Photo Researchers, Inc.)

is not recommended for melanoma since a wide margin is necessary. The other issue is that melanoma cells are more difficult to detect on frozen tissue examination as used in the Mohs technique. Mohs technique needs to be tested further before it can be recommended for melanoma treatment. . . .

Aldara Cream

Aldara cream is a synthetic substance used for treating common skin warts and basal cell carcinoma. The substance in Aldara cream activates dendritic skin cells to produce interferons and other cytokines that may activate a strong local immune response against the melanoma cells. The reaction looks and feels like an inflammation on the skin, which reddens. The melanoma either turns into a scab and sloughs off, or is absorbed by the body. Although it is still experimental, there is some evidence that Aldara cream may be useful for the treatment of small, thin melanomas. More research needs to be done to see exactly how effective Aldara cream is; the approach also prevents pathologic review of the specimen. If Aldara is beneficial in further clinical testing it may play a role in selected cases of small melanoma lesions. . . .

FAST FACT

The Skin Cancer Foundation reports that melanoma is the second most common form of cancer for individuals aged fifteen to twenty-nine.

It is so important to find melanoma when it is still small. Early diagnosis can mean complete eradication of the melanoma by simple surgical excision. Constant vigilance, including monthly self-examination and regular dermatology screening, can lead to successful treatment for most melanomas.

New Developments in Skin Cancer Research

Guide4Living

Skin cancer research, like other cancer research, is advancing every day. New possibilities and ideas are being generated on a regular basis. In the following selection the authors discuss some of these new concepts. Immunotherapy, including tumor necrosis factor, or TNF, is currently being looked at as a companion treatment to chemotherapy. Antibodies, or proteins in the body that destroy foreign cells, are being studied for their effectiveness in recognizing and affecting cancer cells. Cancer vaccines are also in the early stages of research, with several different avenues currently being explored. Also covered in the article are warnings against miracle cures and unproven cancer remedies. Guide4Living is an independent, online health information provider.

Research into treatments and cures for skin cancer are advancing every month. At any one time there [are] dozens of clinical trials testing one new therapy or another.

SOURCE: "Skin Cancer Research and Trials," Guide4Living.com, 2008.

It can be quite bewildering for someone newly diagnosed with melanoma as some research trials offer real hope while others are more a case of trial and error.

Gene Therapy and Other Developments

Gene therapy is among the latest techniques now being tested to treat melanoma as well as other cancers. It involves putting selected DNA into cancer cells to produce proteins which cause the cancer cells to die, make them more susceptible to toxic drugs or stimulate the immune

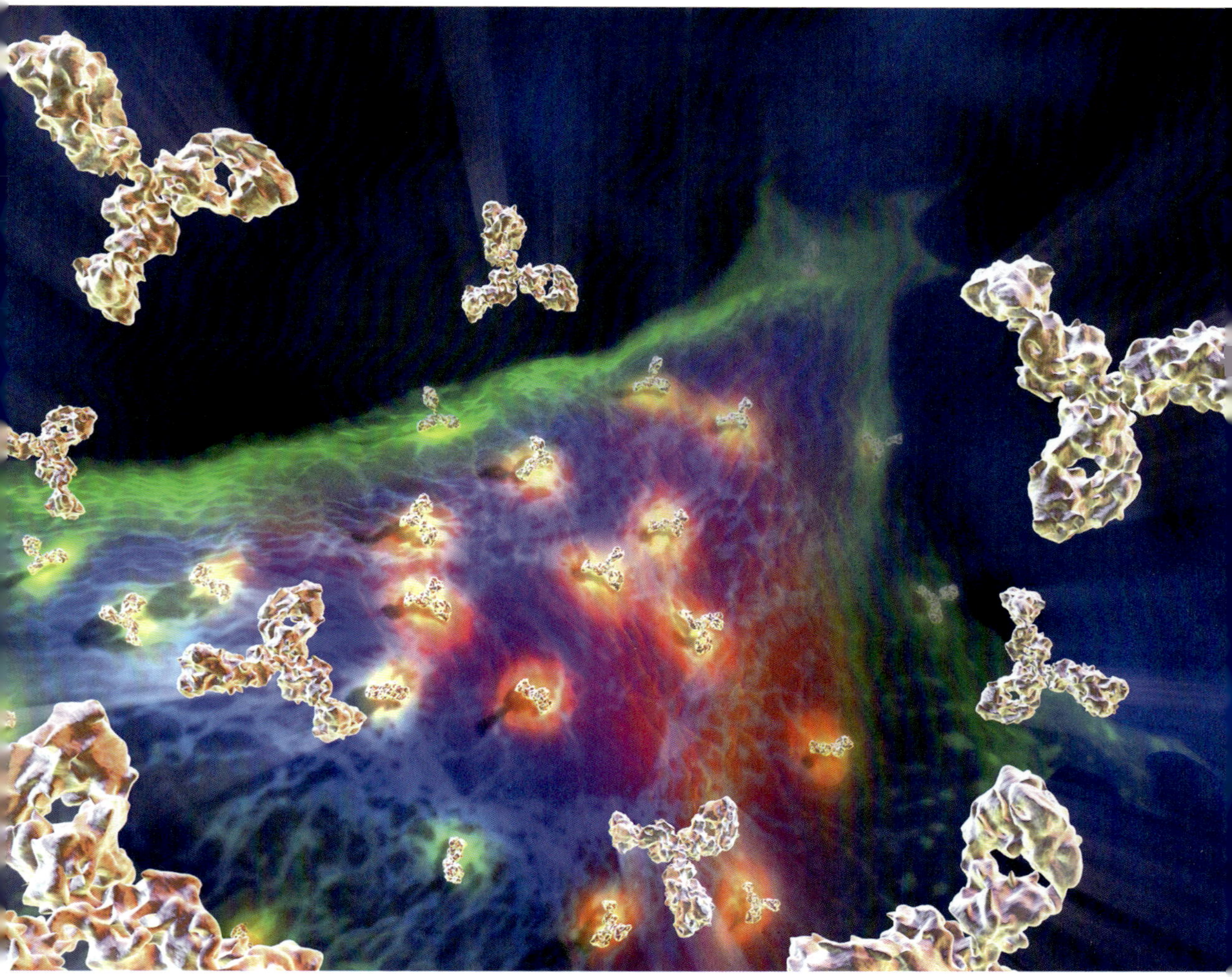

Y-shaped bio-engineered antibodies approach a cancer cell. The antibodies are engineered to attack and kill cancerous cells without affecting other cells in the body. (Hybrid Medical Association/Photo Researchers, Inc.)

system to attack the harmful cells. Although clinical trials are under way this is still very much at the experimental stage and as a possible treatment for melanoma gene therapy is still many years distant.

Immunotherapy is under close investigation at the moment. It involves using proteins naturally produced by the body—interferon and Interleukin-2—to boost the immune system and attack the cancer cells. Both proteins have been found to shrink the melanoma in stages 3 and 4. . . .

Tumour Necrosis Factor (TNF) is another immunotherapy being trialled together with chemotherapy. It is normally used on a limb that has already been treated for melanoma using a technique called regional limb perfusion. The affected limb has its blood supply isolated for a short time during which chemo drugs and TNF are pumped into the area to destroy the cancer cells. It is very experimental and the jury is still out on its effectiveness.

Antibodies that recognise certain cancer cells are currently being produced in laboratories (antibodies are basically proteins which attach themselves to bacteria or viruses in order to destroy them). Researchers are looking at attaching these antibodies to chemotherapy or radioactive molecules to deliver them straight to the cancer cells in the hope of killing them off.

> **FAST FACT**
>
> Nearly 10 percent of all U.S. cases of melanoma occur in California, according to the Los Angeles–based Angeles Clinic and Research Institute.

Cancer Vaccines

And then there are cancer vaccines, although research into this is still in the very early stages. Studies are currently under way to discover whether the laboratory-produced vaccines GM2-KLH and QS21 are effective in helping the immune system fight cancer cells. The vaccines are produced by taking melanoma cells from the patient. They are then treated with genes to help produce proteins

How a Vaccine Works

A vaccine is a preparation of killed microorganisms or living, weakened organisms that is injected into the bloodstream. Cells in the blood produce antibodies that attack the foreign cells in the vaccine. Memory cells are left behind that produce a quick response against the same disease.

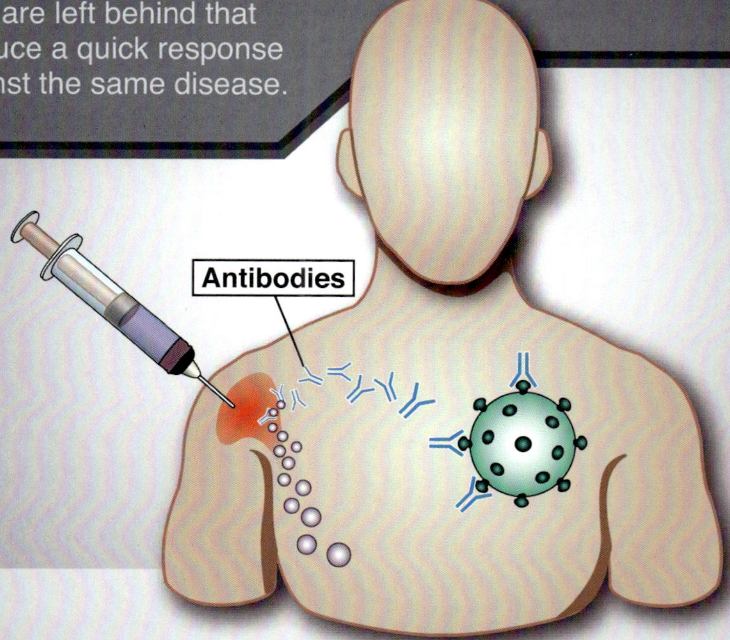

Taken from: Access Excellence, "Making Vaccines," the National Health Museum, 2009. www.accessexcellence.org.

which are already part of the immune system. The cells are treated again with radiation to stop them growing and injected back into the patient to stimulate the immune system and destroy untreated cancer cells. Initial results in small trials have been promising but the likelihood of a vaccine as a cure is still a long way off.

New advances are being made in chemotherapy drugs. Temozolomide, which is successful in treating brain tumours, is now part of a clinical trial to treat melanoma.

Miracle Cures Should Be Treated with Caution

There are always going to be the quack doctors out there offering so called cures and treatments. Trawl the internet and you'll find "miracle" creams made from buffalo testicles claiming to vanish melanomas and pills made from herbal remedies to stop the spread of the disease.

Some people claim these "alternative" remedies work—every advert is accompanied by a glowing testimonial. But health professionals will tell you that such unproven therapies should be treated with caution and conventional treatment should never be stopped suddenly for one of these dubious cure all remedies.

CHAPTER 2

The Controversial Side of Skin Cancer

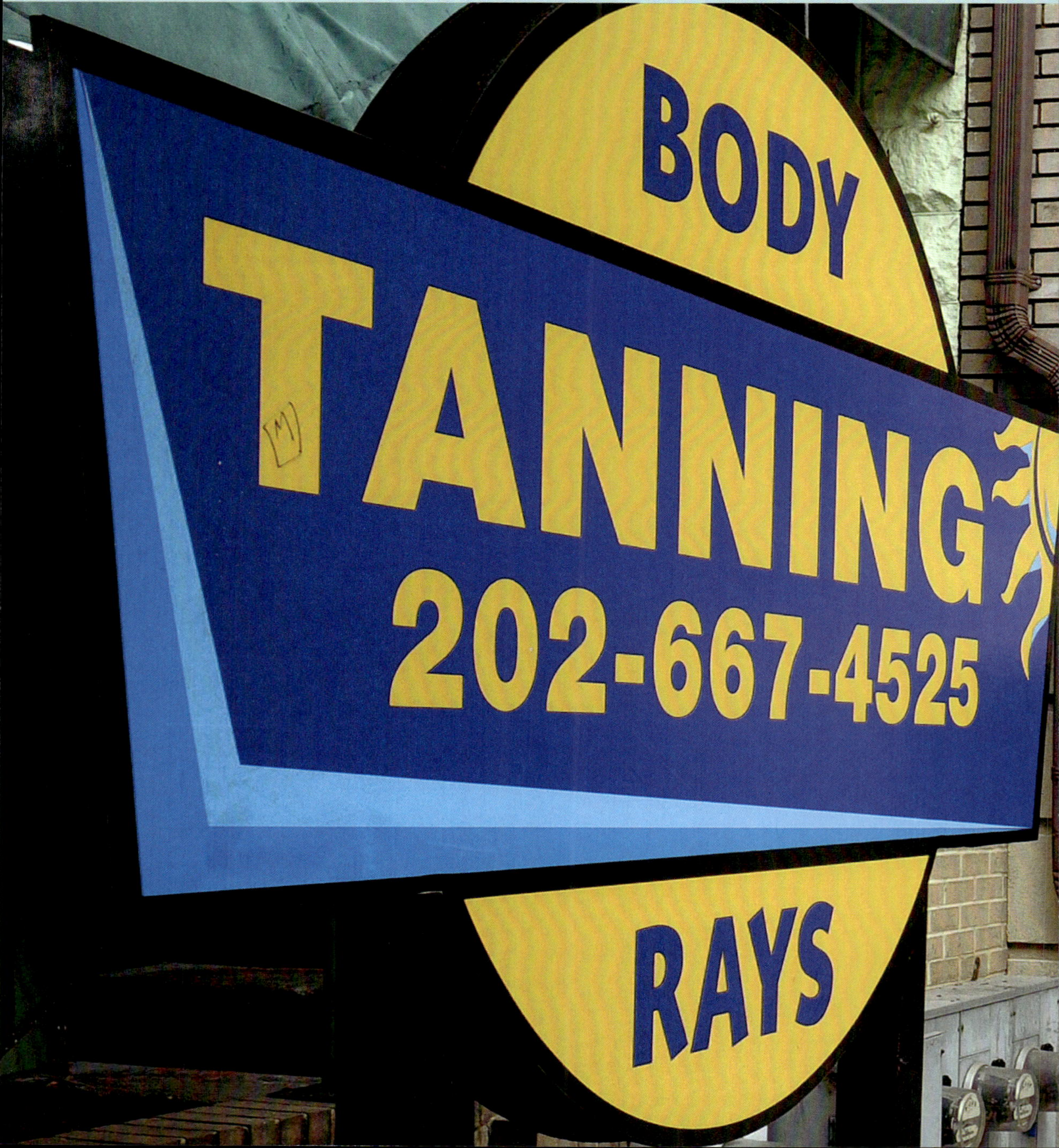

Tanning Beds Are Detrimental to Your Health

Adam Voiland

In the following article reporter Adam Voiland talks about his experiences researching tanning salons and the effects of artificial tanning. According to the author, studies done in the last decade have shown an increasing correlation between indoor tanning and skin cancer. People who use tanning salons have been shown to be as much as two and a half times more likely to get skin cancer as people who do not tan. The question of controlled tanning versus uncontrolled outdoor tanning is also argued, with overall sun exposure being key. Vitamin D and the release of endorphins are also discussed. Voiland is a science and medical writer currently working for the National Aeronautics and Space Administration.

Bronzing agent? Horizontal bed or vertical booth? Eleven thousand or 22,000 watts? Eight minutes or 12? Shopping for a tan isn't for the indecisive, I realized

SOURCE: Adam Voiland, "It's Indoor Tanning Season, but Watch Out," *U.S. News & World Report*, November 15, 2007.

Photo on facing page. Whether tanning salons and tanning devices cause skin cancer is the subject of much controversy. **(Roger L. Wollenberg/ UPI/Landov)**

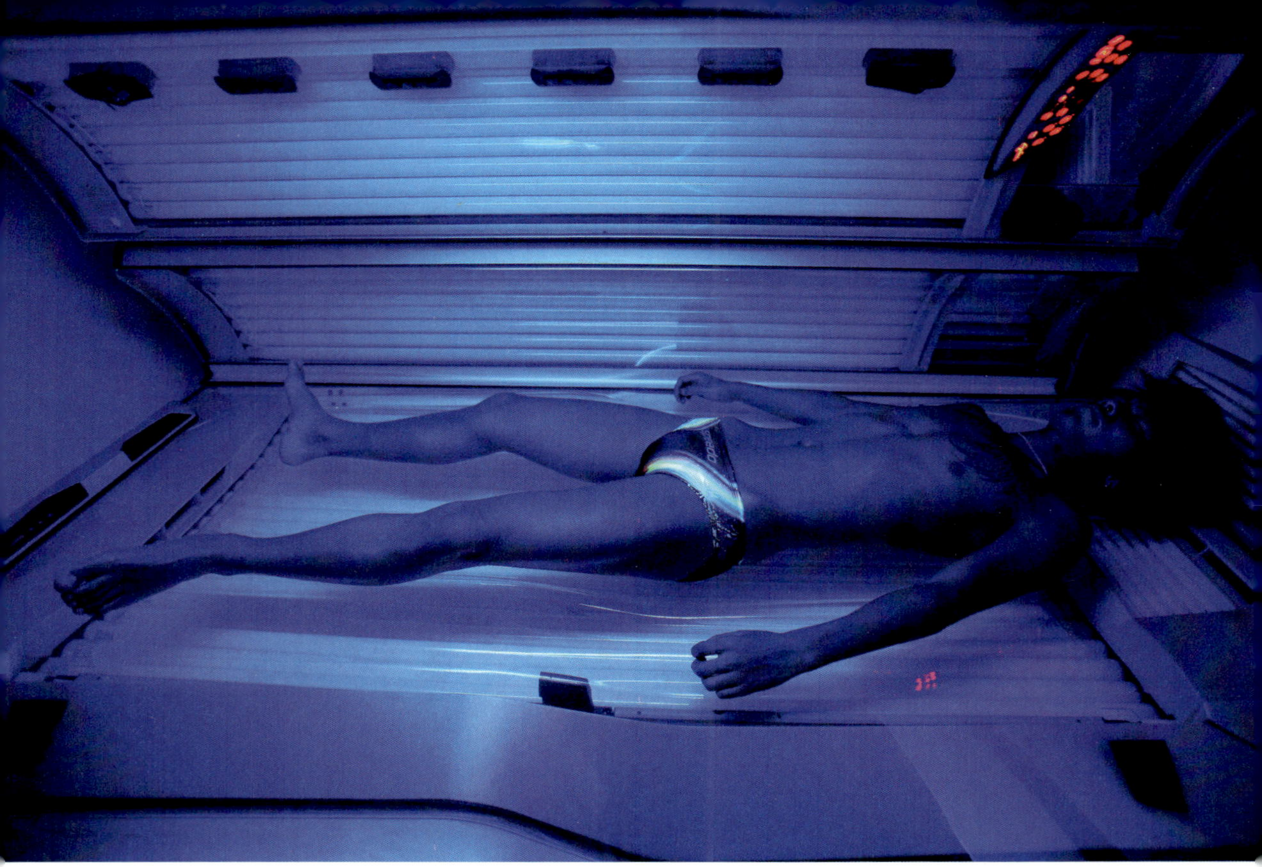

Every year, 30 million people, many of them teenagers, get an indoor tan. Some doctors think that this may be one reason that the rate of skin cancer is skyrocketing. **(Nir Elias/Reuters/Landov)**

during a recent visit to a Solar Planet tanning salon in Washington, D.C. On the advice of the receptionist, I ended up in "The Orbit," a horizontal tanning bed, which looks something like a cross between a coffin and a clam shell and boasts 48 bulbs that produce 11,000 watts of ultraviolet A and B light. After disrobing and applying eye guards and tanning lotion, I eased onto its transparent surface and pulled the lid down around me.

Had I not just spent the day interviewing indignant dermatologists about the wisdom of doing this, it's unlikely I would have noticed the inconspicuous warning label on the Orbit's lid. "Repeat exposure may cause premature aging of the skin and cancer," it said. Hmmm. The fact that lots of people don't appreciate the risks is a big and growing problem, dermatologists argue: Some 30 million people seek an indoor tan yearly, many of them teenagers. And rates of skin cancer are skyrocketing. Melanoma, for example, the deadliest type of skin cancer, has increased more than 690 percent since 1950. And between 2005 and 2006 alone, the rate increased 9 percent. These concerns prompted Congress and the president to pass a law in September [2007] requiring the Food and Drug Administration to consider whether the current warnings on equipment are enough to get the job done.

The Link Between Cancer and Tanning

What are the risks? Reams of new data have come out in the past decade highlighting the link between tanning salons and skin cancer, says Henry Lim, the vice president of the American Academy of Dermatology. One 2002 study by researchers at Dartmouth Medical School found indoor tanners were 2.5 times as likely to get squamous cell carcinoma and 1.5 times as likely to develop basal cell carcinoma as people who didn't tan; the study didn't analyze melanoma rates. Another report from Norway and Sweden followed women who regularly used tanning beds for eight years and found they had a 55 percent greater chance of developing melanoma than those who didn't.

> **FAST FACT**
>
> Blue Cross and Blue Shield of Michigan reports that women who use tanning beds are 55 percent more likely to develop malignant melanoma than women who do not use them.

Some tanning salon advertisements make the case that indoor tanning is a safer option than outdoor tanning because it is more controlled. Many dermatologists find that claim difficult to accept. The fact is that ultraviolet light from tanning beds damages skin in the same way that outdoor ultraviolet radiation does. So it isn't necessarily a matter of one source of UV light being healthier than the other, they say. Rather, the key risk factor is overall cumulative exposure. And the convenience of tanning salons is upping exposure for many people. Moreover, new high-pressure sunlamps emit doses that can be as much as 15 times that of the sun, according to the American Academy of Dermatology.

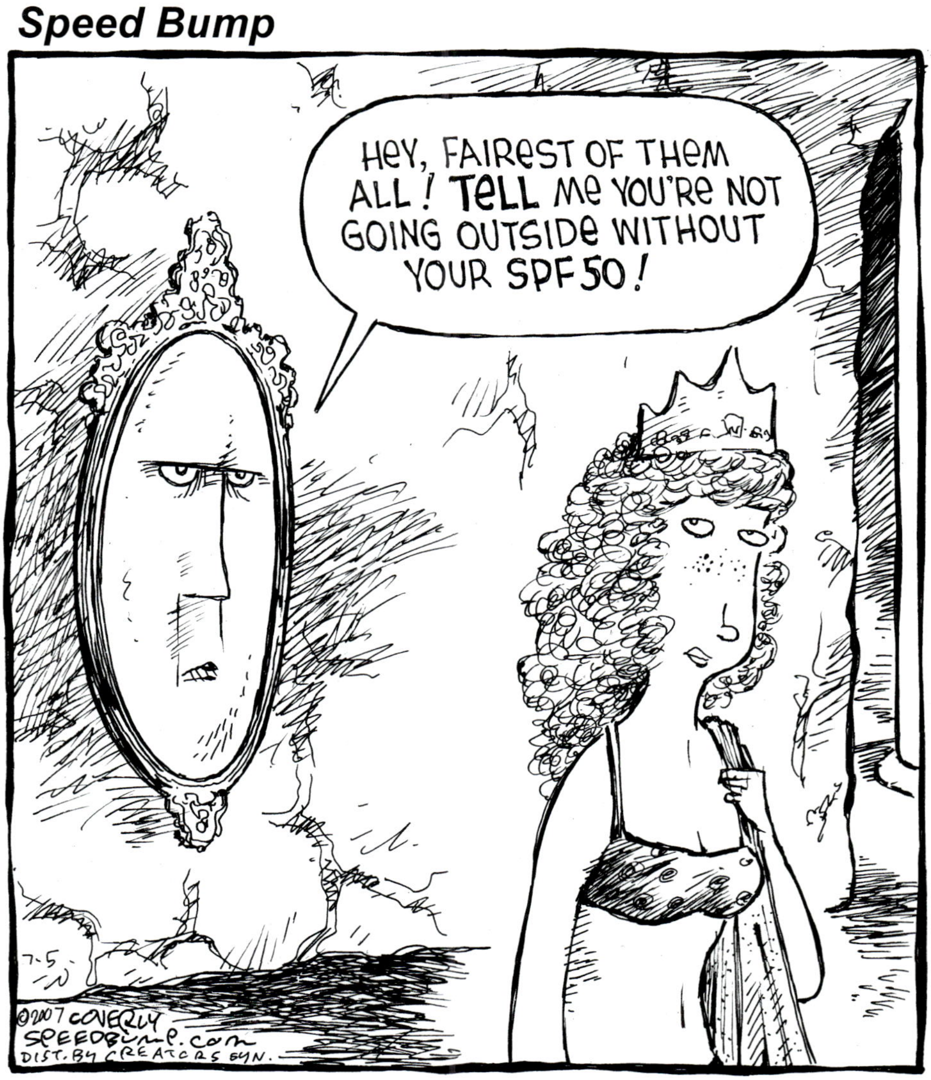

The Benefits of Vitamin D

Not surprisingly, the Indoor Tanning Association, a trade group that represents the tanning industry, counters with the possible benefits of producing extra vitamin D. They point to the work of researchers like Michael Holick of Boston University (who has received funding from the association), suggesting that getting significantly more than 200 international units of vitamin D a day, the current government recommendation for people under 50, can help ward off a host of maladies such as diabetes, cancer, and even the flu. Dermatologists think it's considerably safer to spend 10 minutes or so a few times a week in the sun and look to fish, milk, and dietary supplements for more.

The Release of Endorphins

A few minutes into the $31 session at Solar Planet, as the warm glow envelops me, I can feel a tingling pleasant sensation coming on. Steven Feldman, a dermatologist at Wake Forest University, tells me this is because basking in ultraviolet light releases endorphins that produce the sensation of pleasure similar to that produced by a runner's high. He's even shown that frequent tanners experience withdrawal symptoms when they're cut off. Yikes. That may help explain indoor tanning's appeal, but I'm sure I won't be coming back anytime soon. Even if the increased odds of *death* due to skin cancer may be small, 1 in 5 Americans will get skin cancer, usually because of light exposure, according to the Skin Cancer Foundation. And I already have a number of moles that make my doctors nervous.

Tanning Beds Are Beneficial to Your Health

All Tanning Beds

In the following selection the positive aspects of tanning beds are discussed. One of the benefits of using a tanning bed is enhancement of an individual's beauty, self-confidence, and mood. According to the author, some studies have shown that using a tanning bed improves mood so much that it can motivate an individual to improve him- or herself in other ways, such as eating more healthfully and exercising. The authors also cover a couple of risks in using a tanning bed, including vision problems and other health issues. Looking at all the factors of tanning bed use is an important part of their use. All Tanning Beds is a tanning advice and information provider.

Tanning beds have been in use for many years, and the controversy continues over whether they should be allowed or they should be banned. There are many pros and cons to using tanning beds, and consumers need to arm themselves with the facts before they decide to use one or to avoid them all together.

SOURCE: "Tanning Beds Pros and Cons," All-Tanning-Beds.com, 2008.

Making an informed decision can be difficult because many times the information you find in regards to them are contradictory. Of course, it depends on who is doing the reporting. Tanning bed manufacturers want you to think that they are very safe and only offer a minimal risk.

Beauty, Confidence, and Mood

Tanning beds offer our society a means of maintaining beauty by having skin that has a beautiful color to it. Ask anyone who has ever gone to the pool with pale, pasty white skin how self conscious they felt. Tanning beds are also very fast and convenient. You can get a deep golden color by spending 10 or 15 minutes of your lunch hour at the local tanning salon. You can do it in the evening as well if it fits your schedule better, so you don't have to worry about trying to get some free time while the sun is still blazing in the sky.

Tanning proponents say tanning gives one self-confidence and can also serve as a relaxing interlude. **(Danny Lawson/PA Photos/Landov)**

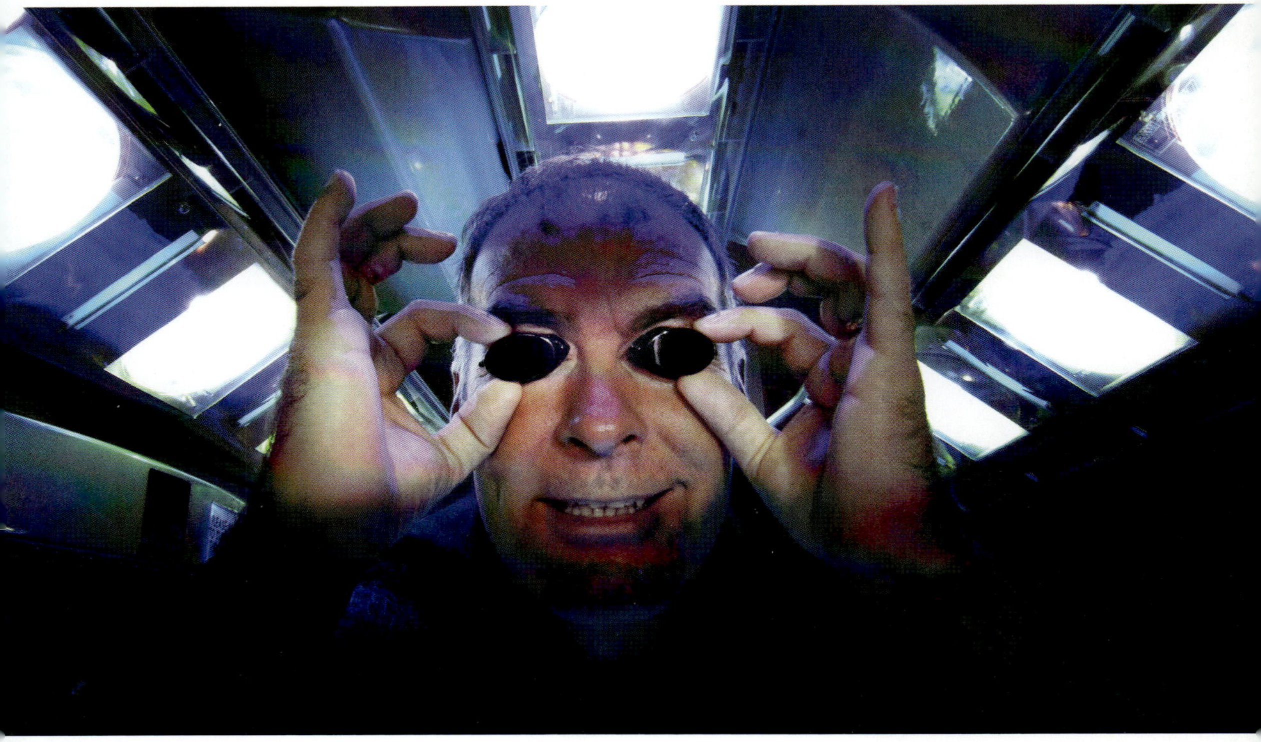

For some people, taking the time to tan gives them amazing self confidence. It also gives them some time in their day to unwind and relax. This is time spent focusing on pampering themselves rather than taking care of someone else. Tanning beds also help the body produce more Vitamin D that helps keep your bones, teeth, and joints very healthy.

In fact, some studies conducted show that a person's mood significantly improves when they use a tanning bed. It makes them feel good about themselves. It can also motivate them to do other things to look good including eat a balanced diet and exercise more often.

Tanning beds are a safer alternative to the harmful rays of the sun. This is because you can get a faster [tan] so you spend less time being exposed to the UV [ultraviolet] rays of the tanning bed than you do direct sunlight. Yet some research indicates that using tanning beds can help the body create melanin which will help prevent the skin from burning when exposed to UV from a tanning bed or direct sunlight.

Mother Goose and Grimm

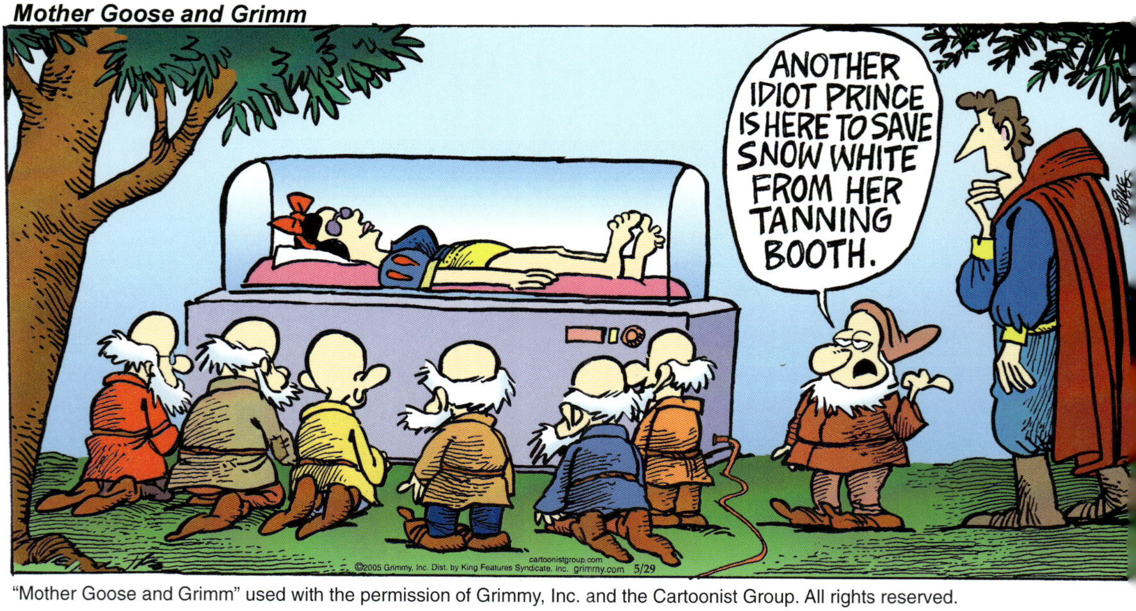
ANOTHER IDIOT PRINCE IS HERE TO SAVE SNOW WHITE FROM HER TANNING BOOTH.

Drawbacks to Tanning Beds

However, research has shown that using tanning beds can have negative effects on your vision, and your health. Tanning beds can lead to your retina or cornea being damaged. They have also been linked to causing cataracts. The UV levels can be up to 100 times stronger than from direct sunlight. The verdict is still out on whether using goggles to protect your eyes while using a tanning bed is sufficient.

Your skin can age rapidly if you use tanning beds for too long of a period of time. The UV rays from tanning beds can also lead to various types of skin cancer just as sunlight can. In some cases it can lead to cancer that cannot be cured and the individual dies. Most people don't realize that tanning beds can be dangerous.

Weighing the Risks

Of course many people take the attitude that nothing is going to happen to them if they use a tanning bed. They may be right, but it is a risk that you really need to think about before you take it.

As long as people are willing to continue using tanning beds, manufacturers and tanning salons will continue to market them. It is important to gather all the facts about tanning beds, both the pros and the cons, so that you can make an informed decision about if using them is worth it or not.

FAST FACT

A study done by San Diego State University found that in many U.S. cities there are more tanning salons than Starbucks coffee shops or McDonald's fast food restaurants.

Indoor Tanning Is Classified as a Cancer Threat

RedOrbit News

In 2009 the World Health Organization (WHO) classified tanning beds as being as carcinogenic as cigarettes and asbestos. In the following news article, a researcher with the International Agency for Research on Cancer (IARC) is quoted as saying that tanning beds can cause cancer of the skin and eye. The researcher notes that this research is supported by previously conducted studies comparing cancer rates for tobacco, alcohol, and asbestos. The article cites researchers who hope that these findings lead to heavier regulation of the tanning bed industry. In addition, the article discusses the reaction of the tanning industry, which disputes the WHO findings. RedOrbit News provides health, science, space, and technology news and information.

The World Health Organization's cancer research agency announced Wednesday [July 29, 2009] that tanning beds and other forms of ultraviolet radiation now rank alongside cigarettes and asbestos as a top-

SOURCE: RedOrbit News, "Tanning Beds Are Cancer Threat," July 29, 2009. www.redorbit.com.

level cancer threat, AFP [Agence France-Presse, a news service] reported.

The International Agency for Research on Cancer (IARC) round soaking up UV [ultraviolet] rays at tanning salons significantly enhances the chances of developing the disease.

Vincent Cogliano, an IARC researcher who led the new assessment, said the use of sunbeds is carcinogenic to humans and causes melanoma of the skin and eye.

Melanoma Risk Greatly Increased

Findings published in the British medical journal *Lancet Oncology* say the risk of melanoma, which is considered the most lethal form of skin cancer, increases by 75 percent when use of tanning devices starts before the age of 30.

However, numerous national health agencies have long warned against using sunbeds.

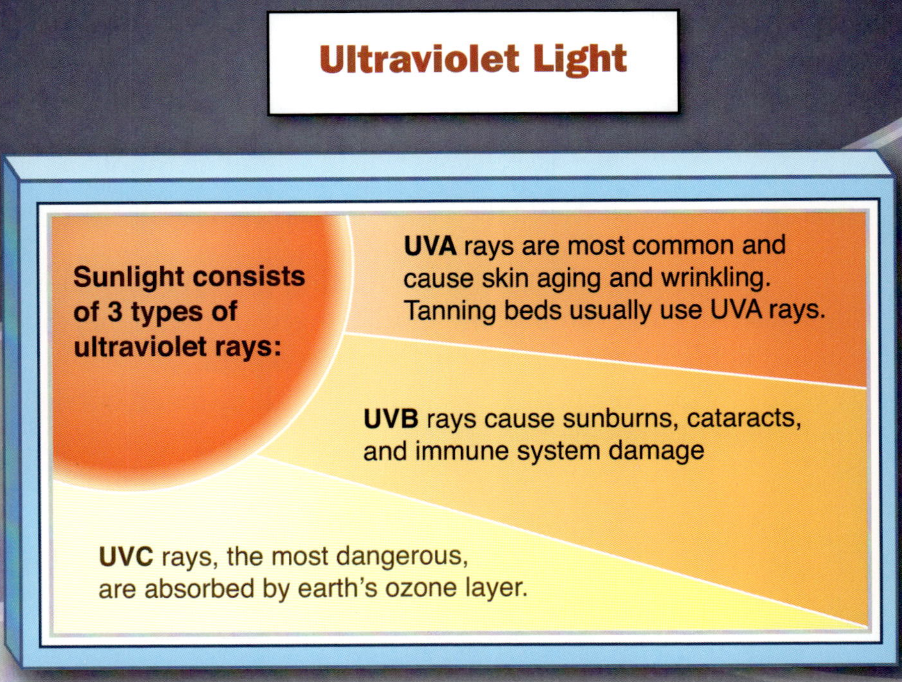

Taken from: Alexandra Bettis, "Does Tanning Cause Skin Cancer?" Vanderbilt University Health Psychology, 2008. http://healthpsych.psy.vanderbilt.edu/2008/TanningCancer.htm.

Animal research and epidemiological studies of cancer rates among humans have provided a high threshold of scientific proof labeling sunbeds a carcinogen comparable to tobacco, asbestos and alcohol.

While it is not the IARC's role to issue recommendations, Cogliano said he hoped the new evaluation would bring attention to the issue.

New Regulations for Tanning Industry

The new research now has many physicians calling for tighter regulations on the multi-billion dollar tanning industry.

Nina Goad, spokeswoman for the British Association of Dermatologists, said they welcome the recognition that sunbeds are carcinogenic.

"It is high time that steps were taken to regulate the industry, to prevent children using sunbeds, and to ensure that sunbeds are subject to health warnings like other known carcinogens," she said.

Meanwhile, George Reuter, the head of France's National Union of Dermatologists, said they have been trying to call the attention of the government to the potential risks for a long time.

FAST FACT

According to *Lancet Oncology*, a British medical journal, the use of tanning beds increases the risk of melanoma by 20 percent.

He told AFP the tubes emitting UV rays vary in intensity and can become more dangerous over time, thus highlighting the need for stricter oversight.

However, neither association is calling for an outright ban of sunbeds.

Reuter said many dermatologists in France simply advise their patients not to exceed 10 sessions in a year.

He believes the solution is to inform the public, not to outlaw sunbeds, adding that those who use the devices to stay tanned year round are especially at risk.

Goad said that people have the right to make their

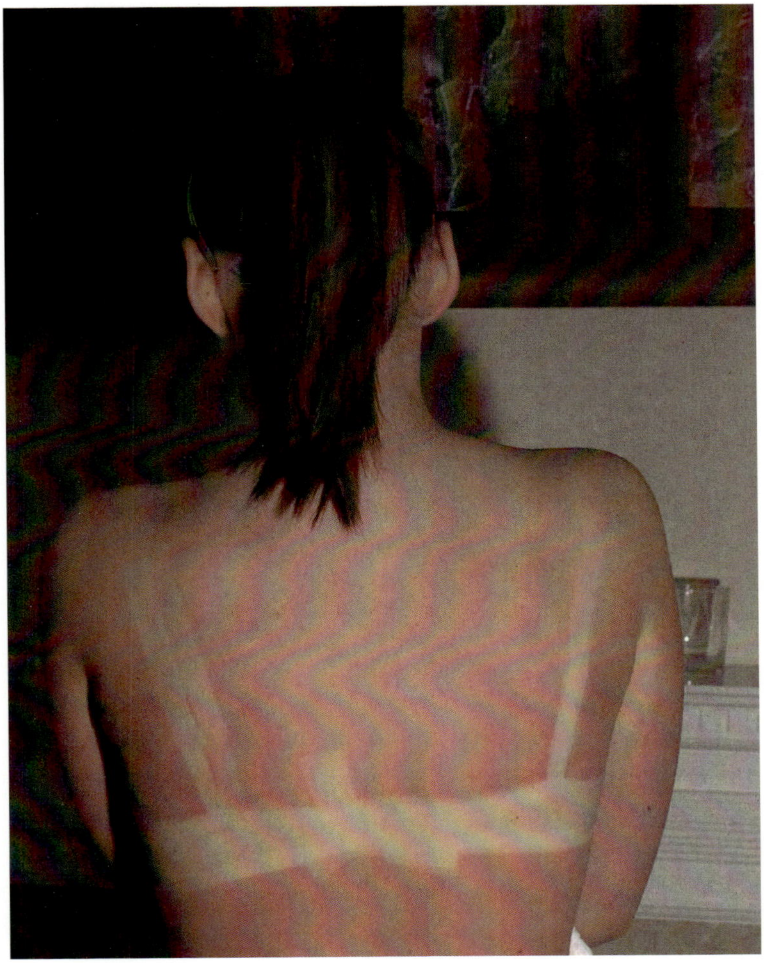

Many teenagers are severely burned in unsupervised tanning beds. (AP Images)

own health choices, noting that other known carcinogens are not banned.

"So I don't think you want to set a precedent with sunbeds," he said.

Tanning Industry Disputes Findings

An industry lobby group based in Britain, known as the Sunbed Association, disputed the IARC's reclassification of tanning devices as carcinogenic to humans.

The group said in a statement: "The relationship between UV exposure and an increased risk of developing skin cancer is only likely to arise where over-exposure—i.e. burning—has taken place."

Kathy Banks, chief executive of The Sunbed Association, a European trade association of tanning bed makers and operators disputed the classification of tanning beds as carcinogenic.

Banks argued it is continuously ignored that there is no proven link between the responsible use of sunbeds and skin cancer, adding that most users of tanning beds use them less than 20 times a year.

Vitamin D from Supplements Is Adequate

L. William Lauro

Vitamin D is an important element in an individual's overall health. Obtained either from the sun or from supplements, the vitamin is showing potential benefits for preventing certain types of cancer. In this selection the author states that vitamin D obtained through fortified foods and nutritional supplements is identical to the vitamin D obtained through direct sun exposure. He also states that any sun exposure over a small amount is wasted because it does not produce any extra amounts of vitamin D. L. William Lauro is a family practice physician and nursing instructor.

"Tanned is beautiful." Do you remember that catchy slogan from the '50's? The folks who developed that slogan, namely the advertising gurus on Madison Avenue, were trying to sell the public tanning oils, coco butter, and UV lamps—all the necessary tools to get

SOURCE: L. William Lauro, "Sunshine, Vitamin D, and Cancer: The Current Controversy," Meridian Magazine, April 22, 2009. www.meridianmagazine.com.

that rich, dark, healthy tan. People were led to believe, through these advertising campaigns (and even some members of the medical community), that a bronzed body, was a healthier body.

But then in the 1960's the data started rolling in that showed the strong association between unprotected sun exposure and skin cancer. The evidence became overwhelming that good old sunshine was a known carcinogen.

At that point my mother started coating her kids with suntan lotion before we went to the beach (we were living in South Florida at the time). And ever since that time my family (and most likely your family, too) has been very vigilant about applying sunscreen before heading out for a day in the sun.

Unfortunately, for many of us who are now middle aged, the tanning excesses of the '50s, '60s, and '70's has created a near epidemic of skin cancer, both non-melanotic (the less serious type) as well as melanotic (the deadliest type of skin cancer).

FAST FACT

A deficiency of vitamin D can cause bone softening, also known as rickets.

But now, despite the volumes of evidence against unprotected sun exposure, a new theory is receiving wide-spread exposure in the lay press: Sun-screens (and sun avoidance) might be eliminating *too much* sunlight from our skins and might therefore be reducing our vitamin D levels, a vitamin that has become popular of late because of its potential anti-cancer benefits.

Does this give us license to head back into the sun and throw our sun tan lotion bottles in the trash? What are we to do?

Let's look at the evidence.

A Brief Review of Vitamin D

Vitamin D was the fourth vitamin discovered and thus named "D" because A, B, and C were already taken (not very original, huh). We all remember from our basic health classes that vitamin D can only be manufactured in our bodies when our skin is exposed to sunshine. It can also be obtained from some of the foods we eat, but in much smaller quantities. This is the reason the food industry supplements many foods with vitamin D.

The creation of vitamin D begins when our skin is exposed to sunshine, first producing an inactive previtamin (vitamin D3) that must undergo further activation in the liver and the kidney. Vitamin D can also be produced by ingesting the inactive precursor vitamin D2 which is found in small amounts in many foods. Both of these inactive pre-vitamins are partially activated by hydroxylation in the liver and then fully activated in the kidney.

And so, unless we eat foods that have been deliberately supplemented with vitamin D, such as dairy products, or unless we take a vitamin pill containing vitamin D each day, or unless we get occasional sun exposure, we may be getting less vitamin D than is optimal for good health.

The Controversy over Vitamin D

But here is the controversy, and it surrounds two points:

1) If we can get vitamin D by simply sun tanning, then why waste our time (and money) taking vitamin D supplements and eating vitamin D–enhanced foods—why not simply get more sun exposure?
2) Is it possible that the vitamin D we consume via supplementation (mainly in the form of vitamin D2) might not be as good as the vitamin D3 that our bodies make naturally when exposed to sunshine?

These questions become even more important when we consider the recent claims that vitamin D might help reduce the chances of getting some forms of cancer. And we already know that vitamin D can help prevent osteoporosis and reduce the risk of multiple sclerosis, type 1 diabetes, and imbalance in the elderly (but only when combined with extra calcium intake). Yes, vitamin D is a hot topic right now.

Two Big Questions

So, in light of these recent studies showing the vast benefits of vitamin D, two questions can be asked: should we be getting more vitamin D in our lives, and, if so, should we be getting it from the sun, rather than through supplements?

These are important questions because the last thing we want to do is unravel all the good that has been achieved these past 30 years through educating the public about the risk of unprotected sun exposure and its link to skin cancer and premature aging of the skin.

To answer the first question, let me tell you about the current recommendations for vitamin D supplementation. For persons younger than age 50, the recommendation is an extra 200 units of vitamin D per day; ages 50–70, 400 units per day; older than age 70, 800 units per day. However, many experts believe these recommendations are too low (some feel that *twice* these amounts are needed, and I happen to agree with this).

By the way, a glass of fortified milk or orange juice (approximately 8 oz) has 100 units of vitamin D in it; and most general multi-vitamin pills have 400 units.

Higher doses of vitamin D, when combined with calcium, have been shown in some studies to reduce colon cancer. We know that osteoporosis is benefited as well. We also know that for some reason an elderly person's balance is helped by extra vitamin D/calcium intake, and thus elderly people who take these supplements have fewer falls. And the exciting news is that Type 1 diabetes and multiple sclerosis may be reduced by extra vitamin D and calcium.

Natural Vitamin D (Sunshine) Versus Supplemented Vitamin D

Which is better? The studies I reviewed all pretty much conclude that naturally obtained vitamin D (via sunshine) *is identical* to that obtained by way of oral consumption (diet and vitamins). There is absolutely no reason to assume you are getting "better" vitamin D, or more vitamin D, by sun tanning. Both vitamin D2 (dietary) and D3 (sunshine) are converted into the same chemical in the liver (partial hydroxylation) and then the kidney (full hydroxylation and activation).

And consider this: When our bodies are exposed to sunshine, vitamin D3 is created, as we discussed above, but it occurs within just a few minutes of sun exposure; *extra sun exposure does not create significantly more vitamin D.* The body has a means by which it caps the production of natural vitamin D via sun exposure so that we

Studies have shown that people can obtain just as much vitamin D from supplements as they can from sunshine. (© **Hermien Lam/ Catchlight Visual Services/Alamy**)

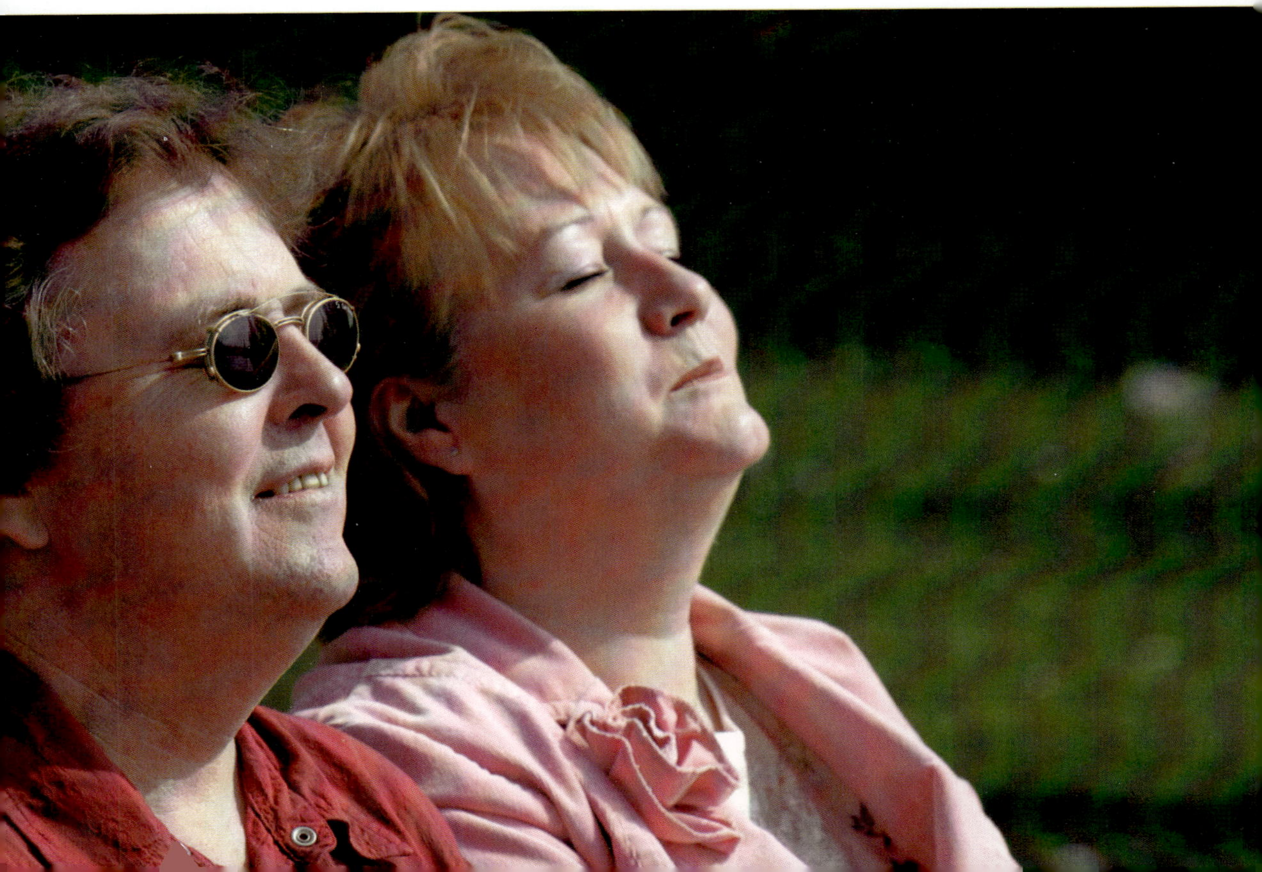

Latitude and Vitamin D Production in the Skin

Except during the summer months, the skin makes little, if any, vitamin D from the sun at latitudes above 37 degrees north (in the United States, the shaded region in the map) or below 37 degrees south of the equator. People who live in these areas are at relatively greater risk for vitamin D deficiency.

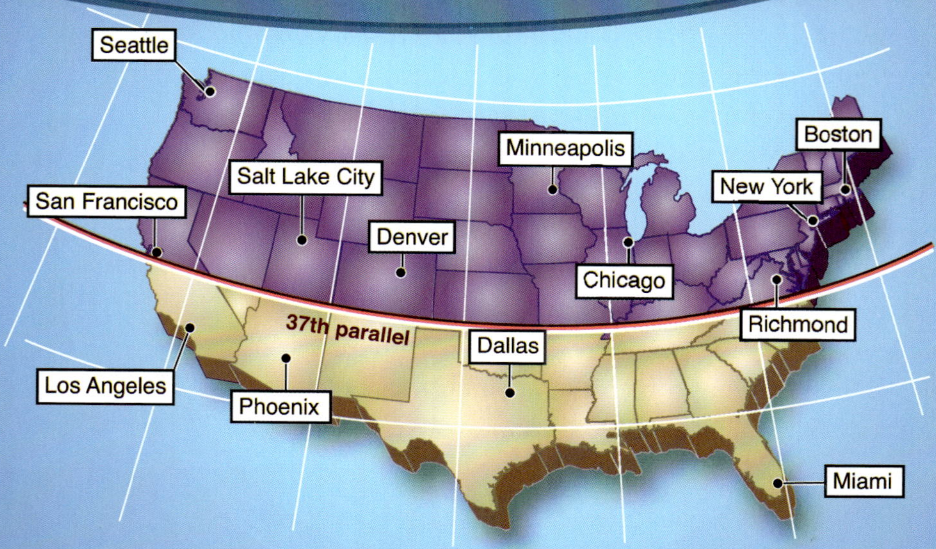

Taken from: *Harvard Women's Health Watch*, "Time for Some More Vitamin D," September 2008.

do not get too much vitamin D (too much can be bad for you). So if you go out into the sun looking for vitamin D production, you will have maximized your skin's ability to make its vitamin D long before you begin to get a pink coloration to the skin (usually about 7–8 minutes of exposure on a sunny day). Any extra sun exposure is a waste of time and exposes you to unnecessary skin cancer risk. As a matter of fact, only 5% of the surface area of the body needs to be exposed to the sun for a brief 7–8 minutes—this is usually accomplished by simply having your hands and face exposed to the sun on a bright day for this brief period of time.

Sun Tan Lotion and Vitamin D

Some scientists have worried that our penchant for using sun tan lotion to reduce the harmful effects of the sun on our skin can reduce our vitamin D production. These experts therefore have speculated that the population might benefit from 10–15 minutes of unprotected sun exposure each day. However, other studies have shown that sun tan lotion is not 100% perfect in eliminating sun penetration of the skin—enough rays still get through to produce significant amounts of vitamin D. So I would not recommend purposely sun tanning without sun tan lotion just to get vitamin D.

Vitamin D and Calcium

Vitamin D alone does not help prevent osteoporosis, nor does it seem to reduce cancer risk. You need calcium as well, something you cannot get from the sun. This argues for supplementation rather than sun tanning as our source of vitamin D. By the way, we should be getting an additional 1000–1500 mg of calcium per day along with our vitamin D supplementation.

Another thing to consider when taking vitamin D, whether one gets it from sunshine or supplements—too much of it can be a problem. Yes, studies have shown that higher doses of vitamin D (along with calcium) can *reduce* the risk of colon cancer, but this same higher dose *increases* the risk of prostate cancer! Nothing is ever as simple as it seems—one cannot just open a vitamin pill bottle and gobble up the pills!

Vitamin D via Sun Exposure Is Not Recommended

Additional vitamin D, along with calcium, seems to have many added benefits. Studies show a decrease in some cancers, as well as a decrease in Type 1 diabetes, multiple sclerosis, osteoporosis, and balance problems in the elderly.

Exposing the skin to sunlight and/or ingesting foods supplemented with vitamin D (or taking vitamin pills with vitamin D added) can provide adequate amounts of vitamin D. However, the amounts of vitamin D that can be produced by sun exposure are limited, it exposes the body to a known carcinogen (sunshine), and it ages our skin prematurely. Also, calcium, which is needed for vitamin D to work its wonders, cannot be obtained from the sun. Therefore, sun tanning cannot be recommended as a source of the additional vitamin D we seek.

But if you do want to have some sun-produced vitamin D, then know this: Vitamin D produced by exposure to the sun can be obtained in significant amounts by as little as a brief 7–8 minute sun exposure of just 5% of the surface area of the body three times a week.

Also, sunscreens do not appear to significantly reduce the amount of sun needed to convert vitamin D in the body—some sunshine still gets through.

Vitamin D from the Sun May Be Important for Health

Associated Press

In the following selection the Associated Press discusses the importance of vitamin D, the sunshine vitamin. Vitamin D is increasingly being shown to help prevent several differing types of cancer, including prostate and lung. Also covered in the article are the drawbacks to obtaining vitamin D via supplements as opposed to the sun. According to the U.S. government, too much vitamin D from vitamin pills can cause unhealthy amounts of calcium to increase in the body. Also cited is the opinion of Michael Holick, professor of dermatology at Boston University, who states that vitamin D from the sun has great advantages over vitamin D from other sources. The Associated Press is one of the world's largest news organizations providing print, photos, graphics, audio, and video.

Scientists are excited about a vitamin again. But unlike fads that sizzled and fizzled, the evidence this time is strong and keeps growing.

SOURCE: Associated Press, "Too Little Sun as Bad as Too Much?" MSNBC.MSN.com, May 23, 2005.

If it bears out, it will challenge one of medicine's most fundamental beliefs: that people need to coat themselves with sunscreen whenever they're in the sun. Doing that may actually contribute to far more cancer deaths than it prevents, some researchers think.

The vitamin is D, nicknamed the "sunshine vitamin" because the skin makes it from ultraviolet rays. Sunscreen blocks its production, but dermatologists and health agencies have long preached that such lotions are needed to prevent skin cancer.

Now some scientists are questioning that advice.

Vitamin D Is Gaining in Importance

The reason is that vitamin D increasingly seems important for preventing and even treating many types of cancer. In the last three months [March–May 2005] alone, four separate studies found it helped protect against lymphoma and cancers of the prostate, lung and, ironically, the skin. The strongest evidence is for colon cancer.

Many people aren't getting enough vitamin D. It's hard to do from food and fortified milk alone, and supplements are problematic.

So the thinking is this: Even if too much sun leads to skin cancer, which is rarely deadly, too little sun may be worse.

No one is suggesting that people fry on a beach. But many scientists believe that "safe sun"—15 minutes or so a few times a week without sunscreen—is not only possible but helpful to health.

A Professor Makes His Case

One is Dr. Edward Giovannucci, a Harvard University professor of medicine and nutrition who laid out his case in a keynote lecture at a recent American Association for Cancer Research meeting in Anaheim, Calif.

His research suggests that vitamin D might help prevent 30 deaths for each one caused by skin cancer.

"I would challenge anyone to find an area or nutrient or any factor that has such consistent anti-cancer benefits as vitamin D," Giovannucci told the cancer scientists. "The data are really quite remarkable."

No Source Is Ideal

The talk so impressed the American Cancer Society's chief epidemiologist, Dr. Michael Thun, that the society is reviewing its sun protection guidelines. "There is now intriguing evidence that vitamin D may have a role in the prevention as well as treatment of certain cancers," Thun said.

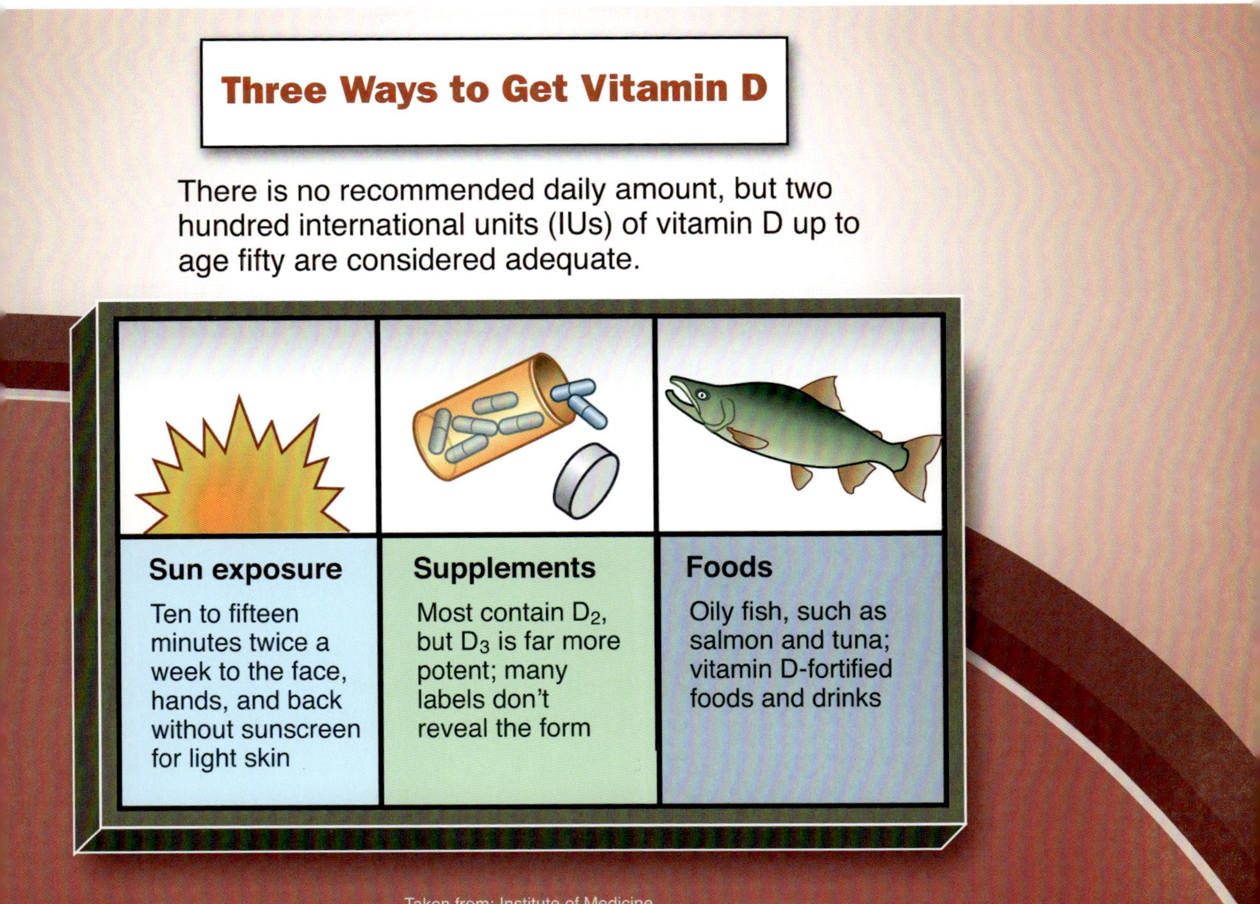

Taken from: Institute of Medicine.

Even some dermatologists may be coming around. "I find the evidence to be mounting and increasingly compelling," said Dr. Allan Halpern, dermatology chief at Memorial Sloan–Kettering Cancer Center in New York, who advises several cancer groups.

The dilemma, he said, is a lack of consensus on how much vitamin D is needed or the best way to get it.

No source is ideal. Even if sunshine were to be recommended, the amount needed would depend on the season, time of day, where a person lives, skin color and other factors. Thun and others worry that folks might overdo it.

"People tend to go overboard with even a hint of encouragement to get more sun exposure," Thun said, adding that he'd prefer people get more of the nutrient from food or pills.

The Difficulties of Vitamin D Supplements

But this is difficult. Vitamin D occurs naturally in salmon, tuna and other oily fish, and is routinely added to milk. However, diet accounts for very little of the vitamin D circulating in blood, Giovannucci said.

Supplements contain the nutrient, but most use an old form—D-2—that is far less potent than the more desirable D-3. Multivitamins typically contain only small amounts of D-2 and include vitamin A, which offsets many of D's benefits.

As a result, pills might not raise vitamin D levels much at all.

Government advisers can't even agree on an RDA, or recommended daily allowance for vitamin D. Instead, they say "adequate intake" is 200 international units a day up to age 50, 400 IUs for ages 50 to 70, and 600 IUs for people over 70.

Many scientists think adults need 1,000 IUs a day. Giovannucci's research suggests 1,500 IUs might be needed to significantly curb cancer.

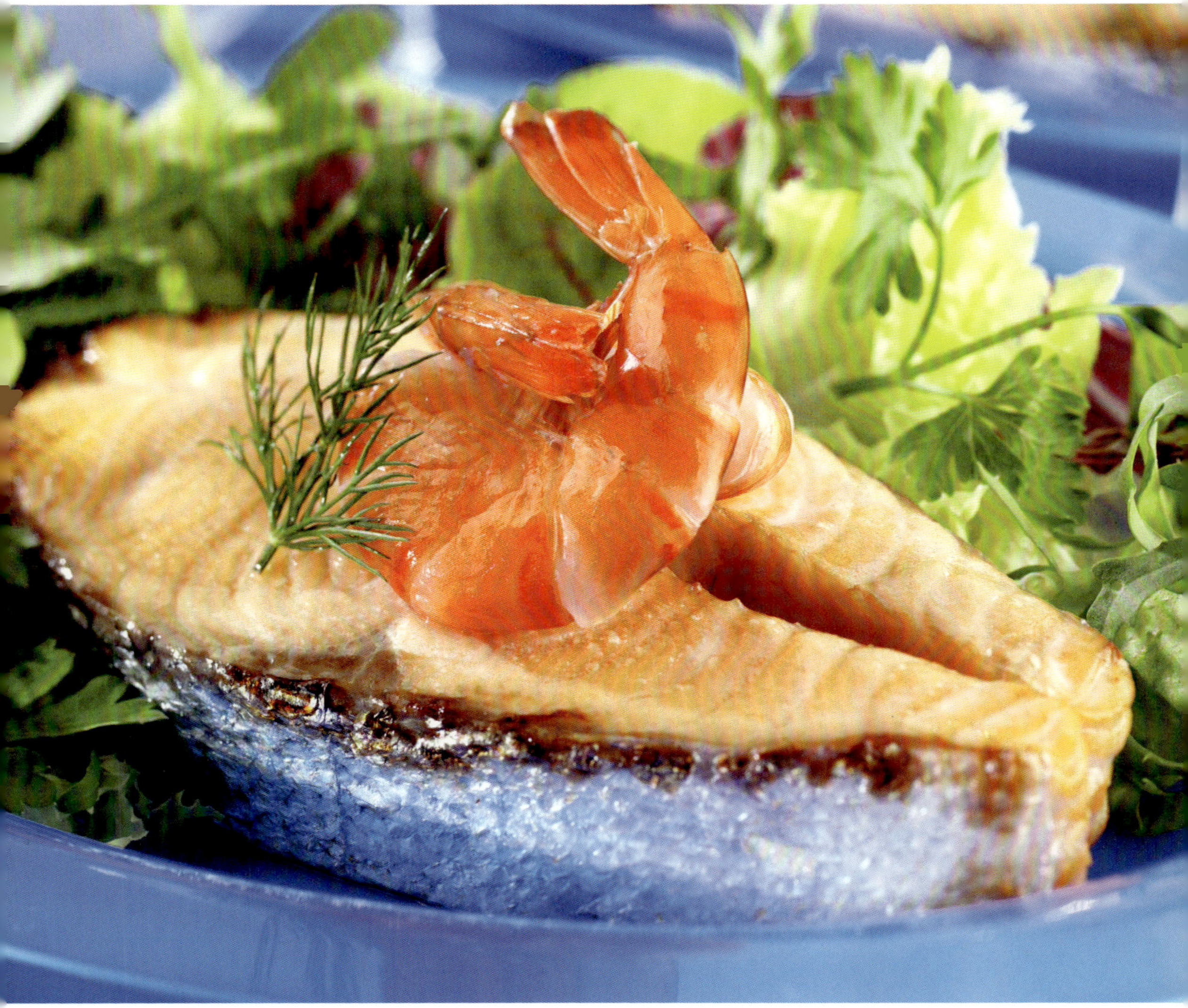

Vitamin D occurs naturally in salmon, tuna, and other oily fish. (© Food and Drink/SuperStock)

How Vitamin D May Curb Cancer

How vitamin D may do this is still under study, but there are lots of reasons to think it can:

- Several studies observing large groups of people found that those with higher vitamin D levels also had lower rates of cancer. For some of these studies, doctors had blood samples to measure vitamin D, making the findings particularly strong. Even so, these studies aren't the gold standard of medical research—a comparison over many years of a large group of people who were given the vitamin with a large group who didn't take it. In the past, the best research has deflated health claims involving other nutrients, including vitamin E and beta carotene.

- Lab and animal studies show that vitamin D stifles abnormal cell growth, helps cells die when they are supposed to, and curbs formation of blood vessels that feed tumors.
- Cancer is more common in the elderly, and the skin makes less vitamin D as people age.
- Blacks have higher rates of cancer than whites and more pigment in their skin, which prevents them from making much vitamin D.
- Vitamin D gets trapped in fat, so obese people have lower blood levels of D. They also have higher rates of cancer.
- Diabetics, too, are prone to cancer, and their damaged kidneys have trouble converting vitamin D into a form the body can use.
- People in the northeastern United States and northerly regions of the globe like Scandinavia have higher cancer rates than those who get more sunshine year-round.

During short winter days, the sun's rays come in at too oblique an angle to spur the skin to make vitamin D. That is why nutrition experts think vitamin D-3 supplements may be especially helpful during winter, and for dark-skinned people all the time.

Use Common Sense

But too much of the pill variety can cause a dangerous buildup of calcium in the body. The government says 2,000 IUs is the upper daily limit for anyone over a year old.

On the other hand, D from sunshine has no such limit. It's almost impossible to overdose when getting it this way. However, it is possible to get skin cancer. And this is where the dermatology establishment and Dr. Michael Holick part company.

Thirty years ago, Holick helped make the landmark discovery of how vitamin D works. Until last year [2004], he was chief of endocrinology, nutrition and diabetes and a professor of dermatology at Boston University. Then he published a book, "The UV Advantage," urging people to get enough sunlight to make vitamin D.

"I am advocating common sense," not prolonged sunbathing or tanning salons, Holick said.

Skin cancer is rarely fatal, he notes. The most deadly form, melanoma, accounts for only 7,770 of the 570,280 cancer deaths expected to occur in the United States this year.

More than 1 million milder forms of skin cancer will occur, and these are the ones tied to chronic or prolonged suntanning.

Brainwashing the Public

Repeated sunburns—especially in childhood and among redheads and very fair-skinned people—have been linked to melanoma, but there is no credible scientific evidence that moderate sun exposure causes it, Holick contends.

"The problem has been that the American Academy of Dermatology has been unchallenged for 20 years," he says. "They have brainwashed the public at every level."

The head of Holick's department, Dr. Barbara Gilchrest, called his book an embarrassment and stripped him of his dermatology professorship, although he kept his other posts.

She also faulted his industry ties. Holick said the school has received $150,000 in grants from the Indoor Tanning Association for his research, far less than the consulting deals and grants that other scientists routinely take from drug companies.

In fact, industry has spent money attacking him. One such statement from the Sun Safety Alliance, funded in part by Coppertone and drug store chains, declared that "sunning to prevent vitamin D deficiency is like smoking to combat anxiety."

"The Skin Can Handle It"

Earlier this month, the dermatology academy launched a "Don't Seek the Sun" campaign calling any advice to get sun "irresponsible." It quoted Dr. Vincent DeLeo, a Columbia University dermatologist, as saying: "Under no circumstances should anyone be misled into thinking that natural sunlight or tanning beds are better sources of vitamin D than foods or nutritional supplements."

> **FAST FACT**
>
> There are three types of ultraviolet radiation: UVA, or long-wave radiation; UVB, or sunburn radiation; and UVC, or short-wave radiation.

That opinion is hardly unanimous, though, even among dermatologists.

"The statement that 'no sun exposure is good' I don't think is correct anymore," said Dr. Henry Lim, chairman of dermatology at Henry Ford Health System in Detroit and an academy vice president.

Some wonder if vitamin D may turn out to be like another vitamin, folate. High intake of it was once thought to be important mostly for pregnant women, to prevent birth defects. However, since food makers began adding extra folate to flour in 1998, heart disease, stroke, blood pressure, colon cancer and osteoporosis have all fallen, suggesting the general public may have been folate-deficient after all.

With vitamin D, "some people believe that it is a partial deficiency that increases the cancer risk," said Hector DeLuca, a University of Wisconsin–Madison biochemist who did landmark studies on the nutrient.

About a dozen major studies are under way to test vitamin D's ability to ward off cancer, said Dr. Peter Greenwald, chief of cancer prevention for the National Cancer Institute. Several others are testing its potential to treat the disease. Two recent studies reported encouraging signs in prostate and lung cancer.

As for sunshine, experts recommend moderation until more evidence is in hand.

"The skin can handle it, just like the liver can handle alcohol," said Dr. James Leyden, professor emeritus of dermatology at the University of Pennsylvania, who has consulted for sunscreen makers.

"I like to have wine with dinner, but I don't think I should drink four bottles a day."

CHAPTER 3

The Personal Side of Skin Cancer

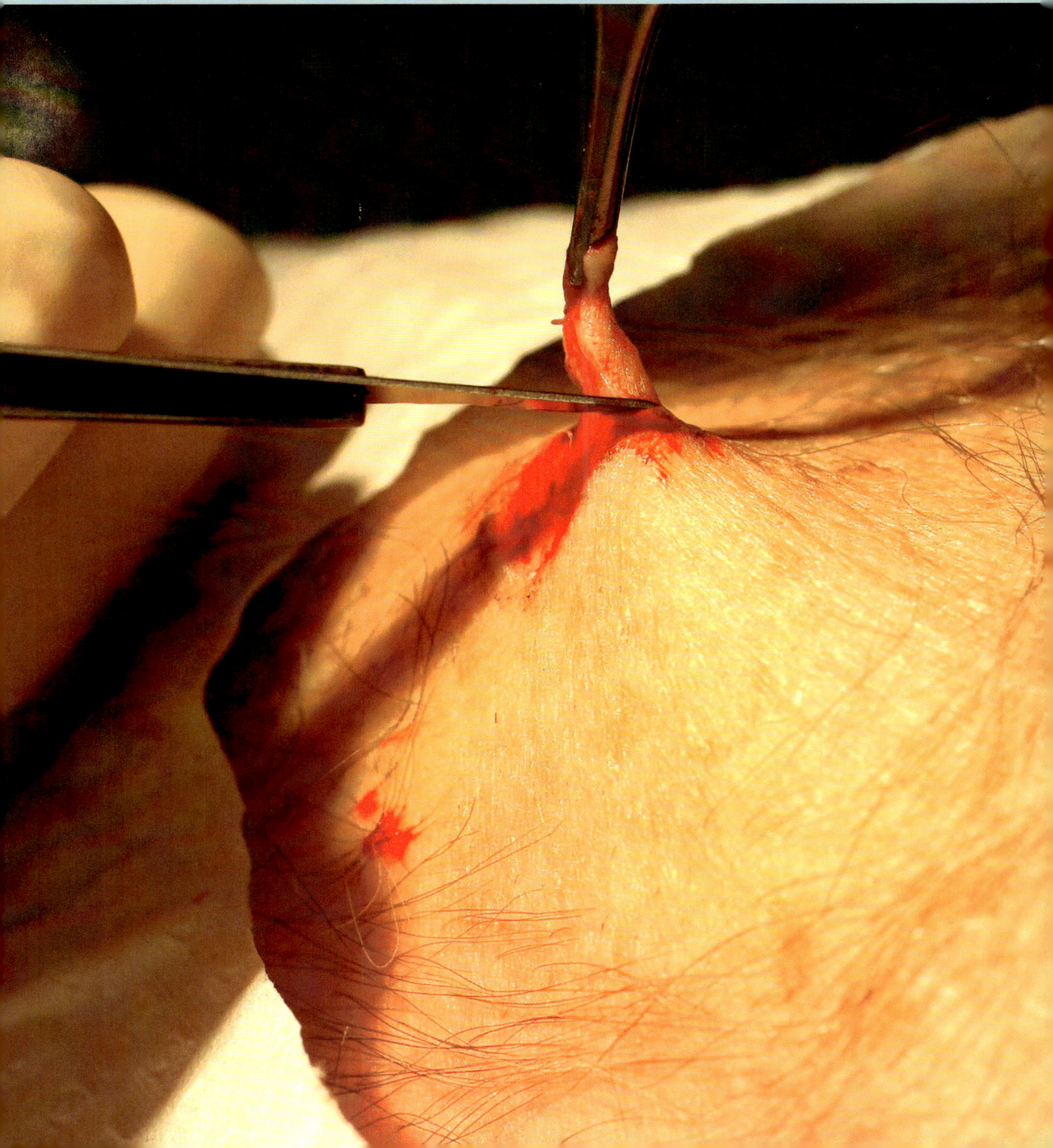

Too Young for Skin Cancer

Jacky Sims

Jacky Sims was fifteen years old when she was diagnosed with malignant melanoma. A resident of the southwestern United States, Jacky was subject to a large amount of sun exposure on a daily basis through sports and regular everyday activities. After her diagnosis she had surgery at the Mayo Clinic in Minnesota to remove a large tumor and then went through a waiting period to find out whether the cancer had spread. After recovering from the surgery, she completely changed her outdoor lifestyle and started working on several different skin cancer outreach programs.

In my hometown of Phoenix, being tan is right up there with having nice clothes and a cool car. And unlike the clothes and the car, it's free. Or so I thought. Even though I wore sunblock, I still had a year-round tan from track, soccer, and swimming.

Photo on facing page. A malignant melanoma skin cancer is surgically removed. **(© cbimages/Alamy)**

SOURCE: Jacky Sims, "Too Young to Get Skin Cancer? Think Again. When I was Only 15 Melanoma Changed My Life," Your Magazine, June 2004. Reproduced by permission.

Malignant Melanoma Diagnosis

In fact, I was heading for the pool last June [2003] when my mom said, "We have to talk." She sat me down and told me that my doctor had found a malignant melanoma. At first I didn't know what she was talking about—I'd never had real health problems. What did she mean, "my doctor"? Then I remembered the mole I'd had taken off my chest a few weeks earlier. There wasn't a lump or anything big, but somewhere under my skin there was a tumor. Tears began rolling down my cheeks as I said, "So does this mean. . . ?" My mom finished the sentence for me: "You have cancer."

The very next day I had an appointment [at] the Mayo Clinic, a world-famous cancer center. The doctor there decided to remove the tumor right away—he didn't want to give the cancer time to spread to my other organs. The urgency terrified me: Was I going to die? When I got home from the clinic, I must have picked up the phone 10 times to call Matt, my then boy-friend. I wanted to tell him the news, but couldn't say the words. So I decided to text him. I burst into tears as I typed: "I have cancer."

Under the Knife

On the drive to the hospital I was wondering why this happened to me. No one in my family had ever had skin cancer. I'd had two moles removed the year before, and neither was cancerous. But thinking about the years of sports in the sun made me sick to my stomach.

By the time we got to the clinic, I was really freaking out. Everything was so white and sterile, and I felt like the doctors were looking at me with a kind of pity. When the anesthesiologist put me under, I was actually relieved.

I woke up a few hours later and glanced down at the huge gash in my chest. For a moment, all I could think about was how terrible the scar would look. Then reality hit and I felt happy to just be alive—and a little anxious.

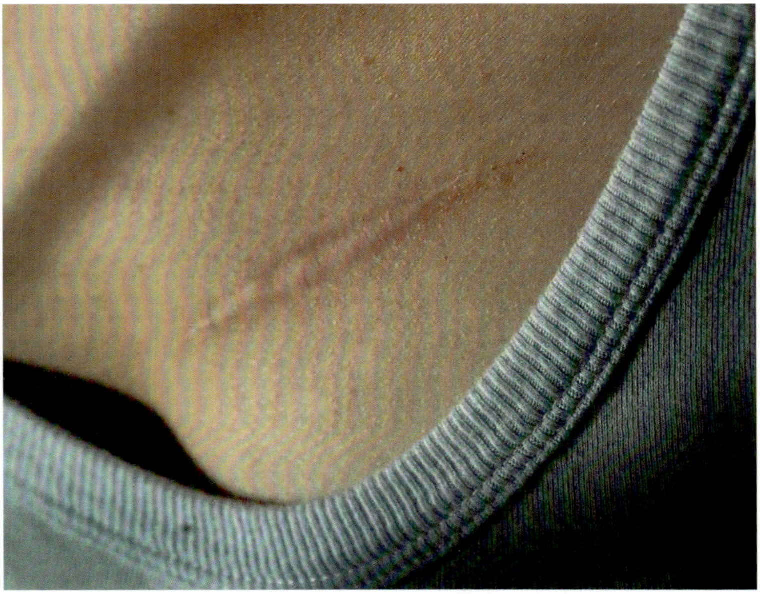

Scarring occurs when doctors surgically remove suspicious melanoma tumors in order to have them biopsied. (AP Images)

The surgeons would biopsy my tumor, and I wouldn't know the results for weeks.

Home from the Hospital

I went home after a few days. To cheer me up, five of my best friends decorated my room and I was showered with cards, flowers, books, and prayers. Knowing that so many people cared about me was comforting, but it didn't stop me from worrying like crazy: there were times when I could feel the cancer inside me, eating away at my body.

Matt took me to a Del Taco for some food, just to get me out of the house. I wasn't totally healed yet—there was a large bandage over my incision—but I still couldn't believe how many people gawked. My 6-year-old neighbor asked innocently what I'd done to myself. I tried to explain that I had skin cancer, but ultimately I simply said I was sick.

Finally, the results of the biopsy came back. The good news was that the melanoma hadn't spread, so I wouldn't need radiation or chemotherapy. Since then, though, I've had five more suspicious cancerous moles removed. That meant surgery and almost daily doctor appointments for a while.

At this point, I'm pretty used to it all. I now have scars on my face, neck, chest, stomach, arm and back, from all the procedures. And I go for full-body checks from a doctor every two months.

Life Goes On

These days, I wake up at 5 A.M. twice a week to do track practice before sunrise, to avoid strong afternoon rays. I'm also working with the SHADE Foundation of America to promote skin-cancer awareness. I make sure their Web site is teen-friendly, and I'm working with them to develop a teen-outreach program. I'd like to think I'm helping other kids avoid what I went through.

> **FAST FACT**
>
> According to San Diego Pacific Oncology and Hematology Associates medical practice, 3 to 5 percent of melanoma patients will find the disease in lymph nodes or other organs without first finding it elsewhere.

The thing that still gets me angry is the common misconception that skin cancer isn't serious. Sometimes, when people hear my story, they'll say stuff like, "Oh, yeah, I had skin cancer. I had a mole removed right here!" That makes me want to scream. Almost 8,000 people will die from melanoma this year. Your chances of developing it are related to your exposure to the sun. So each time you go into a tanning booth or lie out [in the sun], try to imagine your mom or dad telling you that you have cancer. I've been there. It's not worth it.

A Rare Kind of Skin Cancer

Robyn Miller

Robyn Miller, a regular tanning bed user, had been asking her doctor for several years about a lump on her back and was repeatedly told it was nothing to worry about. When the lump became painful, she had it removed and was diagnosed with a rare kind of melanoma. Several additional surgeries followed to keep the cancer in check. She is still undergoing excision procedures whenever another lump appears. Miller explains that she also has a son seriously ill with heart disease and that they battle through surgeries and recoveries together.

Nothing to Worry About

My story begins November 16, 2001. I have had a lump in the center of my back for a number of years—if I were to guess, at least five. Each time I was at the doctor for whatever reason, I would have them check it out just to make

SOURCE: Robyn Miller, "Skin Cancer Personal Stories: Robyn Miller," Guide4Living, January 2005.

sure it was nothing to worry about. Each time I was told not to worry, it was most likely a [lipoma, a benign tumor composed of fatty tissues].

By the summer of 2001 I noticed that this lump had become much larger and somewhat painful. When sitting at work, it would bother me against my chair back, so I decided to have it removed. My doctor sent me to a plastic surgeon who removed it under sedation in December

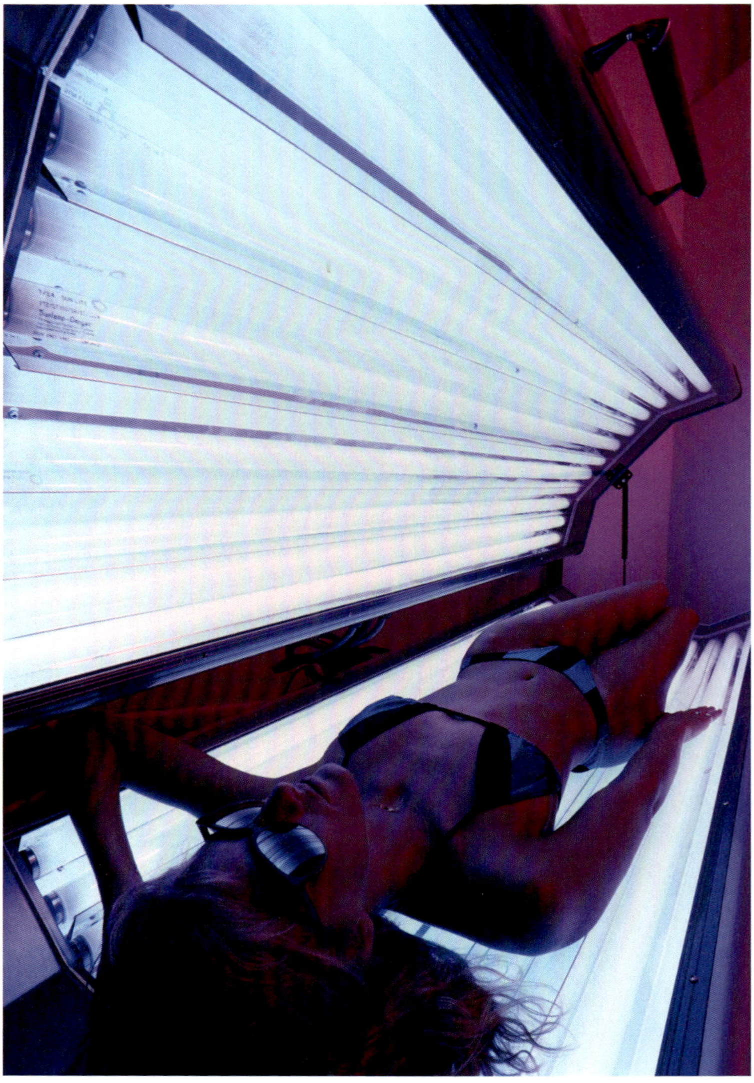

An avid tanner for years, author Robyn Miller was diagnosed with melanoma on her back. Her radiologist believed tanning beds played a large role in the development of the cancer. (© **Chuck Mason/Alamy**)

2001 and I was called into his office about a week later with the results.

The pathology labs in the Lehigh Valley had difficulty identifying the specimen. It was sent to the Armed Forces Labratory in Washington who identified it as a Malignant Blue Cell Nevus (a rare form of cancer that they placed in the melanoma category). I consulted with a radiologist at that time to talk about radiation; however she suggested that a further wide excision was necessary and would be quicker than radiation.

I was an avid tanning bed user for years. I would usually stop from November until February but would tan the rest of the time. The radiologist said that the use of the tanning beds certainly played a large role in accelerating the size and condition of what may have just been a [lipoma].

A Second Surgery Is Performed

In February 2002 my second surgery included a wide excision with skin grafting off my leg and a sentinel lymph node mapping that showed them [where] to remove lymph nodes from under my arms. I am very happy to say that the cancer had not spread to my lymph nodes. This surgery was well tolerated; however there were still margins involved.

At this time I went to see an oncologist in my area who said he did not feel comfortable treating me because he had never seen this kind of cancer before. That evening I went home and researched all the main cancer hospitals in the US on the web. To make a long story short, I ended up choosing Sloan Kettering Cancer Center in New York. I have been going there ever since March 2002.

Repeated Cancer Surgeries Are Necessary

Since March of 2002 until today [January 2005], I have had five more surgeries due to the spread of this cancer (all on my back). They all form as a lump and are always deep when finally recognized on the surface. I am currently recovering from my last re-excision one week ago. I go to get stitches out next Thursday in NY [New York]. The Sloan Kettering Cancer Center is wonderful but two hours away from me, so each visit is an exhausting one until I return home.

FAST FACT

A study published in *Pediatrics*, the journal of the American Acadamy of Pediatrics, found that the children of skin cancer victims were more likely to report frequent sunburns than those without a family history of the disease.

As of today, there is no other treatment available for melanoma other than finding problem areas and cutting them out. It isn't until they spread to major organs or lymph nodes, that there are more forms of aggressive treatment.

Looking back on my past and not knowing what my future holds with this cancer, I would have stayed out of the tanning beds and just walked around a little paler than everyone else. Now when I go to the shore, I need to be covered with sun lotion and under an umbrella. A sun burn in any area now is even more dangerous. I can't change what has already happened to me but perhaps I could change the minds of others that are considering using ultra violet light to make them look temporarily good.

Three Women and Skin Cancer

Medical News Today

In the following selection three different perspectives on melanoma are presented. In the first story a mother talks about her shock when she found out her daughter had terminal melanoma. After her daughter's death Colette Coyne made melanoma awareness her personal crusade. In the second story Natalie Johnson, Miss Utah 2002, talks about losing her twenty-one-year-old brother to melanoma. When she won her title, Johnson used that platform to increase skin cancer awareness. In the third story a farm girl, Robin Lawrence-Broesch, from southern Indiana discusses her years-long battle with melanoma. Working at a local cancer center, Lawrence-Broesch uses her own experiences and scars to help educate people about the dangers of skin cancer.

Studies show that more than 1 million new cases of skin cancer will be diagnosed in the United States this year [2005], with an estimated 10,590 deaths expected. But what these statistics don't reveal are the personal stories

SOURCE: Medical News Today, "Personal Perspectives in Skin Cancer," May 3, 2005. www.medicalnewstoday.com.

of people affected by skin cancer—from the young mother who tanned obsessively as a teenager and now is battling recurring melanoma, to the family members of skin cancer victims who lost their lives and find inspiration by helping others learn how to prevent this potentially deadly condition.

Speaking today [May 2005] at the American Academy of Dermatology's (Academy) Melanoma/Skin Cancer Detection and Prevention Month news conference, three women affected by skin cancer shared their experiences and how they have funneled their pain and grief into raising awareness about this preventable condition.

Colette Coyne

For Colette Coyne's daughter, Colette Marie Brigid Coyne, her battle with melanoma started four years after noticing a change in a mole that was partially removed when she was 22 years old. At age 26, surgery was performed to remove the remaining portion of the mole, which was not diagnosed as melanoma.

Unfortunately, that diagnosis changed four years later when Colette experienced soreness under her arm. In May 1998, Colette learned that four inoperable tumors under her arm were to blame, but this time the diagnosis was melanoma. Colette underwent unsuccessful chemotherapy and by August 1998 the melanoma had spread to her liver, lungs, bones and brain.

"When we were told that Colette's cancer was terminal, we were shocked. She died two and half months later," said Colette's mother, Colette Coyne. "But Colette never wanted to be a cancer victim. She faced her death courageously and spent her remaining time sharing her love with family and friends. Her brave fight and her concern for family enabled us to get through this horrible time and

FAST FACT

The American Academy of Dermatology reports that almost every hour, one American dies from melanoma.

inspired us to make melanoma awareness our cause, our tribute to her."

Through the support of family, friends and coworkers following her death in 1998, the Colette Coyne Melanoma Awareness Campaign (CCMAC) was founded. It is dedicated to increasing public awareness of skin cancer and working to change attitudes and behaviors when it comes to tanning and sun exposure. On April 4, 2005, CCMAC's local efforts to impose tanning regulations for minors paid off as the Nassau County Legislature unanimously passed a new law restricting teenagers' access to tanning salons. Known as the Colette Coyne Skin Cancer Prevention Law, teens under age 18 will need parental permission to use a tanning bed and those under age 16 will need to be accompanied by a parent. Tanning salons also will have to post signs warning patrons about the health hazards of tanning and begin keeping records of all tanning sessions.

"While we are grateful for what has been accomplished, there is still much work to do on the legislative front to establish laws regulating tanning salons and ensuring that only dermatopathologists examine skin biopsies," said Coyne. "Colette's spirit is with us, strengthening us as we strive to help other families in their fight against melanoma."

Natalie C. Johnson

When Natalie C. Johnson lost her 21-year-old brother, Eric, to melanoma and a rare germ-cell tumor within two months of his diagnosis, Johnson and her family quickly learned how their family history put them at an increased risk of skin cancer.

"Growing up in northern California, my family was generally aware of the risks of skin cancer and took sun safety precautions most of the time," said Johnson. "But it is our physical characteristics—blonde hair, fair skin, blue eyes—

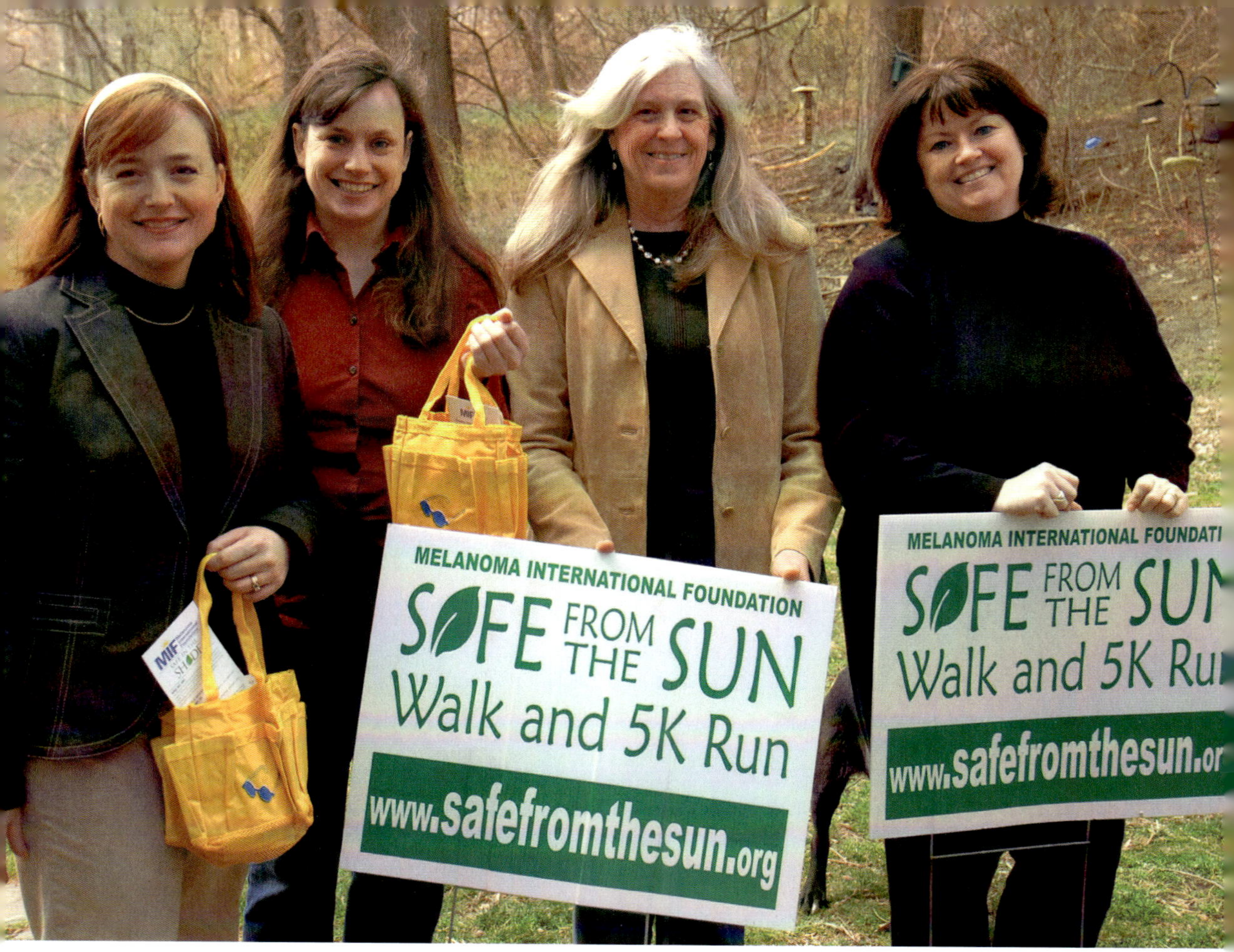

Many skin cancer survivors are involved in organizations that promote skin cancer awareness. (**AP Images**)

coupled with our genetic predisposition to develop multiple abnormal moles that I believe put our family at an increased risk for developing this deadly condition. While my mother and aunt both developed basal cell carcinoma and my grandfather had actinic keratoses, my brother succumbed to melanoma before he even had a chance to fight."

After months of grieving, Johnson decided to use her brother's tragedy as a way to fight for those at risk for skin cancer and began a crusade in her home state of Utah to raise awareness and teach others how to recognize the warning signs of melanoma. Through her work at the High Risk Melanoma Clinic at the Huntsman Cancer Institute in Salt Lake City, Johnson taught patients the ABCDs of melanoma, assisted in the clinic's yearly free skin cancer screenings, and participated in lobbying efforts at the Utah State Capitol that led to the allocation of $4 million to the clinic for cancer research and treatment.

In 2002, her involvement in skin cancer education became her platform when she won the Miss Utah title of the national Miss America Organization. Through her efforts, Johnson was able to broaden her work statewide and reached more than 500,000 Utahns with her skin cancer prevention message.

In April 2003, Johnson co-founded the Cancer Crusaders Organization (a.k.a. the Utah Cancer Crusaders), a non-profit service organization aimed at providing effective cancer education for Utah's college-age population. Recently, the organization launched the "Only Skin Deep?" campaign to provide colleges with an in-depth skin cancer prevention curriculum and worked with the governor of Utah in getting an official declaration signed at the state capitol recognizing and adopting Johnson's Skin Cancer Awareness ribbon.

"I am so fortunate to be able to honor my brother's memory by spreading the word about skin cancer prevention," said Johnson. "Skin cancer doesn't have to be a death sentence, but it requires all of us to educate ourselves on the risks and take precautions in the sun every day of our lives."

Robin Lawrence-Broesch

As a farm girl raised in southern Indiana, Robin Lawrence-Broesch spent much of her time out in the fields on hot sunny days and was part of the generation that used baby oil and iodine to get a good tan. After graduating high school, she started competing in bodybuilding competitions and began using tanning beds to sport the dark tan that was so popular in this sport. Lawrence-Broesch loved being tan and seized every opportunity to be outside in the sun and planned every vacation to sunny destinations.

But Lawrence-Broesch's sun-worshipping lifestyle soon caught up with her.

In March 2002 she learned that she had melanoma and in the three years since her original diagnosis, Lawrence-Broesch has had a total of 19 biopsies—five of which were melanoma.

"The question I kept asking myself was 'Why me?'" said Lawrence-Broesch. "After looking back on my life, I realized I had only myself to blame. But I can honestly say that when I was growing up, I knew very little about the dangers of tanning or the threat of skin cancer. It's so ironic that my pursuit of a healthy, active lifestyle was what would eventually come back years later to threaten my life."

Working as the director of marketing at the Evansville Cancer Center in Evansville, Ind., Lawrence-Broesch realized that she could illustrate the ugly side of tanning by showing her own personal battle scars from melanoma to help educate others. She has conducted more than 100 presentations in middle schools, high schools, universities and for the public reaching more than 12,000 people. A familiar figure at health fairs and community swimming pools, Lawrence-Broesch distributes educational information about skin cancer and free sunscreen.

Through her work in educating others about skin cancer, Lawrence-Broesch has met several people with melanoma—including some who weren't as fortunate to have the same outcome as hers.

"I met a 24-year-old mother of two who died two months after being diagnosed with melanoma," explained Lawrence-Broesch. "I had a chance to talk to her before she passed away and videotaped our conversation to share her story with kids to let them know that the only difference between her and me is that I'm alive because of early detection."

Coaching with Cancer

Jim Calhoun

University of Connecticut men's basketball coach Jim Calhoun has more than one national title to his name. He also has skin cancer. In 2008 he had a lump removed from his jaw, followed by radiation treatments. This skin cancer episode followed a previous finding of skin cancer in his cheek. In the following essay Calhoun talks about the two skin cancer episodes and also about his fighting prostate cancer. He discusses his feelings on how cancer affected him, his family, and his outlook on life.

When I first learned I had skin cancer, just like everybody else, I was a little bit nervous. That "C" word is not anybody's favorite word, and understandably so. The first time it was in my face, and it was squamous cell, which was a small, self-contained cell, right in my cheek. The doctors were going to take it out,

SOURCE: Jim Calhoun, "Sharing Miracles: Cancer," SharingMiracles .com, February 25, 2009.

and quite frankly, it didn't seem like that big a deal at the time. I was still a little bit nervous, obviously, because of the word "cancer", but the word "contained" was a much better word. And that situation was resolved rather quickly.

A Second Episode

The second time, however, was entirely different. The doctors told me that the squamous cell that was contained had somehow or other ended up in my lymph node on my neck, and at the end of the 2008 season, I started to feel something . . . a bump . . . in my neck, and this little internal pimple or bump started to grow . . . and grow . . . and grow. After about three weeks, I went back to the doctor and he said it was nothing, just an inflamed lymph node, he was pretty sure, and he didn't think it was going to be a big problem.

> **FAST FACT**
>
> According to the American Academy of Dermatology, approximately 64 percent of individuals who died from melanoma in 2008 were men.

Well, I went home and the bump was soft, just like the doctors said it would be. It was moveable, just like they said it would be. But, it continued to grow, so I went back to the hospital. At that point, I had what they call a skinny scan—nothing more than taking a needle, putting it into the lump, and doing pathology from there. Three days later they called me and said: you have cancer in your lymph node.

My wife and I went home, sat down and started thinking, this is serious stuff. The doctors couldn't give me answers at that point in time, but I did know I had cancer and immediately had to start thinking about how I was going to handle it, and my wife and I had to talk to each other about the rest of our lives. And as you can well imagine, that night was a very difficult one for me.

Four days later, I had a cat scan and the good news it revealed was that the cancer was just located in one spot on my neck. That was the good news. But, the other open question was: had it metastasized? And they could only know that by going inside and getting it. We were able to schedule my surgery five days later. I had 63 stitches from my ear to my Adam's apple. They cleaned out the tumor and removed 37 lymph nodes. I had a heck of a scar, let me tell you.

Prostate Cancer

With the prostate cancer diagnosis, I was a little bit young at the time to be having it, but, regardless, got to know about the disease very quickly, and the doctors started talking about different solutions. I said: look, it doesn't belong in my body, and I'm willing to fight, just like I fight anything on the court, like I've fought all my life, and I want this out of my body as quickly as possible. Five days later I had a radical prostatectomy, and thank God everything worked out fine. I missed 14 days and went back to

With his physician by his side, University of Connecticut head basketball coach Jim Calhoun (right) talks to members of the press about his battle with skin cancer. **(AP Images)**

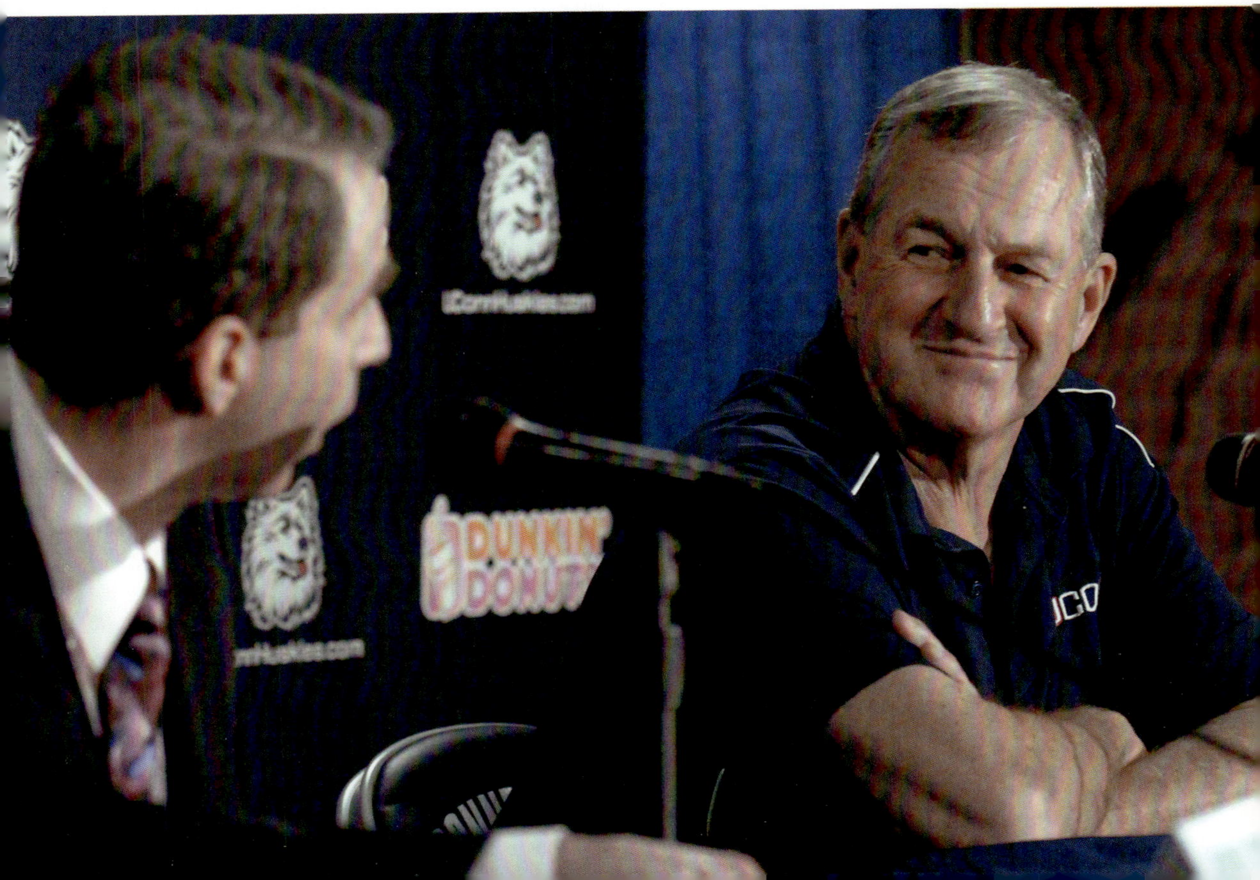

coaching. They say it's a record, but trust me, I didn't feel that great on the bench for the next six months. I paid a price for it.

No one in my family—I have four sisters and a brother—ever had cancer before, so it was really kind of shocking to have cancer come into our house. The most difficult part of the whole thing was feeling vulnerable—feeling that something could attack me that I had no control over. And then, quite honestly, the other difficult part was going public. It was hard going public. No one really wants to talk about their weaknesses, and I guess the male ego says that you don't want to be weak or be attacked. And I was weak . . . and I was being attacked. And I had to admit it. But I felt I had an obligation because I was in a position to affect many, many people. And as it turns out, according to the American Cancer Society in Connecticut, record numbers of people came out for PSAs [prostate cancer tests], which put a smile on my face.

Nothing in Life Is Guaranteed

In my opinion, we don't have a script in life that is written for us. We write every single chapter of our lives. That's why we have to make every day a special challenge. I like challenges—they stimulate you, and motivate you. And when you're afflicted with something like cancer, remember, there are so many other people who love and care about you. And you have an obligation to make sure that you attack that, too.

So from me to you, let's go get 'em.

GLOSSARY

actinic keratosis A patch of scaly, rough skin that can develop into squamous cell carcinoma.

basal cell carcinoma A slow-growing form of skin cancer that originates in the cells of the epidermis. The cells of this cancer look much like the basal cells of the skin. This type of skin cancer is the most common type, has a high rate of recurrence, and tends to spread locally on the skin.

benign tumor A noncancerous growth of tissue.

biopsy The removal of tissues or cells for examination by a pathologist to check for disease or damage.

cancer A disease in which normal body cells grow and multiply without any normal controls. As they multiply, the cells form a tumor, or cancerous growth.

carcinogen A substance that can cause cancer.

carcinoma A malignant cancer that begins in the skin or the lining of an organ.

cell An individual unit of protoplasm. Every animal and plant is made up of one or more cells.

clinical trial A research program using real patients that evaluates a certain type of treatment, drug, or procedure. Clinical trials often lead to widespread use of improved methods of treatment. These studies are also referred to as clinical studies.

congenital Something that exists at the time of birth.

cutaneous Relating to the skin.

dermatologist A physician specializing in the study and treatment of the skin and its associated ailments.

dermis The layer of skin directly below the epidermis. Capillaries run through this layer; it also contains hair follicles, nerve cells, and sweat glands.

dysplastic nevus An abnormal mole, usually irregular in shape, size, and color.

epidermis The outermost layer of skin.

excision The removal of an entire area of skin.

keratinocytes The basic cell type of the epidermis. These are produced by basal cells in the inner layer of the epidermis.

lesion A growth or patch of skin that does not resemble the surrounding tissue.

malignant Cancerous.

melanin A pigment that helps protect the skin from ultraviolet light. Melanocytes increase melanin production in response to sun exposure.

melanocytes Skin cells that produce the pigment melanin. These types of cells are found in the basal layer of the epidermis and can develop into skin cancer.

melanoma This is the most dangerous type of skin cancer, and melanomas often spread to other organs in the body.

metastasize To spread from one area or region of the body to another.

Mohs surgery The removal of cancerous tissue, layer by layer until cancer-free tissue is found.

mole A pigmented spot on the skin.

nevus A mole.

oncologist A physician specializing in the treatment of cancer.

pigment A substance that gives color to skin, hair, and eyes.

precancerous lesions Changes in the skin that are not cancer but could become cancer in the future.

prognosis The outlook for recovery from a disease.

radiation therapy Cancer treatment that uses X-rays or other kinds of radiation to kill or stall the growth of cancer cells. There are two types of this treatment: external, which uses a machine to bombard the cancer from outside the body; and internal, which uses a radioactive substance (usually seeds, wires, or catheters) to dispense radiation from inside the body.

remission The decrease or disappearance of the symptoms of a disease.

risk factor An environmental or other variable that increases a person's chance of developing cancer or other diseases.

SPF (sun protection factor) A scale developed to rate the degree of protection provided by sunscreens.

squamous cell carcinoma Skin cancer that originates in the squamous cells of the epidermis. This skin cancer has a thick, scaly, and irregular appearance.

squamous cells The main structural cells of the epidermis.

subcutaneous Occurring in the subcutis.

subcutis The innermost layer of skin. The layer of fat and connective tissue attaches the skin to tissue beneath, and the blood vessels in this layer feed the capillaries of the dermis.

tumor An abnormal growth of tissue. A tumor can be malignant or benign.

UV (ultraviolet) rays Waves of radiation energy that are emitted by the sun. There are three types of UV rays: UVA and UVB, which can penetrate the ozone layer; and UVC, which cannot. UVB is the stronger of the two that can penetrate the ozone layer, but UVA can pass deeper into the skin than UVB.

CHRONOLOGY

B.C.	400	Hippocrates uses the terms *carcinos* and *carcinoma*, which leads to the word *cancer*.
	300	Galingal, a type of ginger root, may have been used to treat skin cancer.
A.D.	500	Tanned skin is very undesirable, and ancient Greek and Roman women use whitening paints as skin lighteners.
	1500s–1800s	Women protect their skin from all possible sun exposure through the use of hats, bonnets, parasols, and gloves. Tanned skin is associated with lower- and working-class women.
	1712	Bernardo Ramazzini publishes *De Morbis Artificum Diatriba*, which describes occupational hazards, including skin conditions of lead miners and other workers.
	1764	The English title of Ramazzini's work, *The Diseases of Workers*, is published.
	1775	British physician Percival Pott finds skin cancer in chimney sweeps. This is the first time anyone documented an environmental agent causing cancer.
	1787	Scottish doctor John Hunter removes a cancerous growth from a patient. Almost one hundred years later, this growth is shown to be melanoma.
	1800s	The Cherokee use red root, a native North American shrub, to treat skin cancer.

1804 Melanoma is discussed as a disease for the first time by French doctor René Laënnec at a medical conference in Paris.

1840 Scientist Samuel Cooper reports that advanced stage melanoma is untreatable.

1872 Kaposi's sarcoma is first described by physician Moritz Kaposi. This cancer, which causes abnormal tissue growth under the skin and in the lining of the mouth, nose, and other organs, will become associated with the AIDS epidemic ongoing since the late 1900s.

1890 Francis Elias Spinner dies of skin cancer in Florida on December 31. Spinner was appointed U.S treasurer by Abraham Lincoln and served in that capacity until his retirement in 1875.

1900 Swedish physician Thor Stenbeck treats and cures a skin cancer patient using small doses of radiation. This process is later referred to as fractionated radiation therapy and will become the basis for present-day radiation treatments of cancer.

1915 Japanese scientist Katsusaburo Yamigiwa reports that coal tar has been shown to cause carcinomas on the skin of rabbits.

1918 Australian dermatologist Norman Paul publishes *The Influence of Sunlight in the Production of Cancer of the Skin.*

1920s Fashion designer Coco Chanel becomes tan during a European trip, and tanning becomes the newest fashion craze.

1928 The first documented sunscreen is introduced in the United States. It contains benzyl salicylate and benzyl cinnamate.

1930 Specific chemicals are found to be carcinogenic, including some of those found in coal tar.

1930s With the advent of color film, being tan becomes a status symbol for Hollywood actors so that they look glamorous in the new medium.

1936 L'Oreal founder E. Schueller introduces the first commercially available sunscreen.

1940s Pharmacist Benjamin Greene develops red petrolatum-based sunscreen to help protect soldiers.

1956 Australian scientist Henry Lancaster discovers a relationship between melanoma and latitude, due to the intensity of the sun. He concludes that sun exposure is a large risk factor in the development of skin cancer.

1972 The U.S. Food and Drug Administration reclassifies sunscreens from cosmetics to over-the-counter drugs.

1974 The SPF numbering system is developed by a Harvard University photobiologist.

1975 The ability to sequence DNA is developed. This leads to identifying abnormal genes that cause cancer.

1977 Johnson & Johnson develops the first waterproof sunscreen.

1978 The FDA first proposes regulations for the use of sunscreen.

1979 The first ultraviolet tanning salon opens in the United States.

1981 Reggae artist Bob Marley dies of melanoma and brain cancer on May 11.

1987 President Ronald Reagan has a melanoma removed from his nose. Six months later the cancer reappears and is removed via Mohs surgery.

1989 A British woman asks to have a mole removed after her dog repeatedly sniffs at it while ignoring all other moles. The growth is found to be melanoma.

1991 The first human gene therapy is attempted for the treatment of melanoma.

1993 Arizona senator John McCain is diagnosed with melanoma.

1996 Armand Cognetta, a Florida-based dermatologist, reports to the National Cancer Institute that his dog George is more than 99 percent effective in detecting skin cancer.

1997 A *Seventeen* magazine surveys finds that two-thirds of teenagers believe an individual looks healthier with a tan. New rule updates for the use of sunscreen are proposed by the FDA.

2000 Arizona senator John McCain is again diagnosed with melanoma. The U.S. Food and Drug Administration reports that not all suntan lotions and preparations contain sunscreen ingredients.

2004 The cost of treating non-melanoma skin cancer for this year is $1.5 billion.

2007 New rules for the use of sunscreen are proposed by the FDA and now include standardized testing methods for sunscreen preparations. More than 1 million new cases of skin cancer are diagnosed in this year.

2008 Monell Chemical Senses Center reports at the 236th American Chemical Society meeting that basal cell carcinoma, the most common form of skin cancer, has a different "scent profile" than normal skin.

2009 The U.S. Food and Drug Administration continues screening new rules for the labeling and use of sunscreens. A new skin cancer diagnosis kit is available for skin self-exams.

ORGANIZATIONS TO CONTACT

The editors have compiled the following list of organizations concerned with the issues debated in this book. The descriptions are derived from materials provided by the organizations. All have publications or information available for interested readers. The list was compiled on the date of publication of the present volume; the information provided here may change. Be aware that many organizations take several weeks or longer to respond to inquiries, so allow as much time as possible.

American Academy of Dermatology
930 E. Woodfield Rd.
PO Box 4014
Schaumburg, IL 60168-4014
(888) 426-3376
www.aad.org

This organization of physicians specializing in care of the skin offers sun care programs, dermatologist referral services, and support groups. It advocates scientific and clinical research, education, and skin care and disease awareness. Brochures are available through its Web site. Its informational Web site SkinCancerNet (www.skincarephysicians.com/skincancernet/index.htm) provides detailed information on all aspects of skin cancer, including prevention, diagnosis, visuals, skin examinations, and risk factors. New releases and pertinent articles are also available.

American Cancer Society
15999 Clifton Rd. NE
Atlanta, GA 30329
(800) 227-2345
www.cancer.org

The American Cancer Society is a nationwide, community-based health organization with over thirty-four hundred local offices. The society's goal is to eliminate cancer as a health issue and to help fight cancer through research, education, patient service, advocacy, and rehabilitation.

American Institute for Cancer Research
1759 R St. NW
Washington, DC 20009
(202) 328-7744
(800) 843-8114
www.aicr.org

This organization concentrates on providing information on cancer prevention, mainly through diet, weight management, and physical activity. It also offers cancer pamphlets for the general public and a cancer resource guide for patients and their families.

American Osteopathic College of Dermatology
1501 E. Illinois St.
Kirksville, MO 63051
(660) 665-2184
(800) 449-2623
fax: (660) 627-2623
www.aocd.org
info@aocd.org

This organization is a specialty college of the American Osteopathic Association. Through its Web site it offers an extensive skin disease database and archived issues of the *Journal of the American Osteopathic College of Dermatology*. Also available is a dermatologist referral service.

Centers for Disease Control and Prevention (CDC)
National Center for Chronic Disease Prevention and Health Promotion
Division of Adolescent and School Health
(800) 232-4636
www.cdc.gov/HealthyYouth
cdcinfo@cdc.gov

This division of the CDC provides detailed skin cancer information geared toward adolescents. Basic facts, risk factors, and prevention are covered, along with programs specifically designed for young people. Individual questions and concerns can be addressed through its Web site and toll-free phone line.

National Cancer Institute
6116 Executive Blvd.
Rm. 3036A
Bethesda, MD 20892-8322
(800) 422-6237
Live help:
www.cancer.gov/help

This government institute, part of the National Institutes of Health, is the principal government agency for cancer research and training. The institute provides detailed information on all types of cancer, and free information is provided upon request. A live help line is also available through its Web site.

National Women's Health Information Center
Office on Women's Health
8270 Willow Oaks Corporate Dr.
Fairfax, VA 22031
(800) 994-9662
www.womenshealth.gov

This government program, part of the Office on Women's Health in the U.S. Department of Health and Human Services, specifically addresses women's health issues through developing health programs, educating health professionals, and disseminating women's health information to the general public. The center has information on more than eight-hundred health topics and offers health publications, statistics, daily news, and calendars of health events. Detailed information on skin cancer, skin care, and skin aging is available.

Skin Cancer Connection
Health Central Corporate Headquarters
2300 Wilson Blvd.
Ste. 600
Arlington, VA 22201
(703) 302-1040
fax: (703) 248-0830
www.skincancerconnection.com

This Web site, one of the Health Central Network of medical sites, provides detailed skin cancer information, references, skin cancer–related resources, news, treatment option information, drug information, and a question and answer message board. Skin cancer updates and information are provided by doctors and other health professionals.

Skin Cancer Foundation
149 Madison Ave.
Ste. 901
New York, NY 10016
(212) 725-5176
(800) 754-6490
www.skincancer.org

The Skin Cancer Foundation concentrates solely on the disease of skin cancer through education, prevention, early detection, and effective treatment methods. Its Web site offers detailed information on the differing types of skin cancer and various prevention methods. Topics associated with skin cancer, such as tanning and vitamin D, are also covered. Brochures, books, CDs, and other informational media are available through the Web site and the toll-free phone line.

FOR FURTHER READING

Books

Lise Alschuler and Karolyn A. Gazella, *"Alternative Medicine" Magazine's Definitive Guide to Cancer*. Berkeley, CA: Celestial Arts, 2007.

Mary Mills Barrow and John Barrow, *Sun Protection for Life: Your Guide to a Lifetime of Healthy and Beautiful Skin*. Oakland, CA: New Harbinger, 2005.

Roy Burdon, *The Suffering Gene: Environmental Threats to Our Health*. London: Zed, 2003.

Bill E. Cham, *The Eggplant Cancer Cure: A Treatment for Skin Cancer and New Hope for Other Cancers from Nature's Pharmacy*. Petaluma, CA: Smart, 2008.

Andrew H. Ko, Malin Dollinger, and Ernest H. Rosenbaum, *Everyone's Guide to Cancer Therapy: How Cancer Is Diagnosed, Treated, and Managed Day to Day*. Kansas City, MO: Andrews McMeel, 2002.

William I. Lane and Linda Comac, *The Skin Cancer Answer: The Natural Treatment for Basal and Squamous Cell Carcinomas and Keratoses*. Garden City Park, NY: Avery, 1998.

Edward F. McClay, Mary-Eileen T. McClay, and Jodie Smith, *100 Questions and Answers About Melanoma and Other Skin Cancers*. Sudbury, MA: Jones and Bartlett, 2004.

Marion Morrie and Eve Potts, *Choices: The Most Com-*

plete Sourcebook for Cancer Information. New York: HarperCollins, 2003.

Catherine M. Poole and DuPont Guerry IV, *Melanoma: Prevention, Detection, and Treatment.* New Haven, CT: Yale University Press, 2005.

Al Sears and Jon Herring, *Your Best Health Under the Sun.* Wellington, FL: Wellness Research and Consulting, 2007.

World Health Organization, *Exposure to Artificial UV Radiation and Skin Cancer.* Lyon, France: World Health Organization, 2006.

Periodicals

Associated Press, "New Treatment Saves Man with Deadly Skin Cancer," *USA Today*, September 23, 2008. www.usatoday.com/news/health/2008-06-19-melanoma-treatment_N.htm?sF=4.

Patrick Barry, "Seeking Genetic Fate," *Science News*, July 4, 2009.

Sharon Begley, "The Post Investigates Cancer Vaccines," *Saturday Evening Post*, September/October 2009.

Samuel Broder, "Preventing Skin Cancer," *U.S. News & World Report*, January 26, 2009. http://health.usnews.com.

Chris Day, "Agency Says Tanning Beds Cause Cancer," *Stillwater (OK) NewsPress*, August 2, 2009.

Kate Devlin, "Family History of Skin Cancer 'Almost Doubles Risk of Parkinson's,'" *Daily Telegraph* (London), February 16, 2009. www. telegraph.co.uk/health/health news.

Sanjay Gupta, "The Vitamin-D Debate," *Time*, May 18, 2009.

Meryl Davids Landau, "Beware of 'Shadow' Diseases," *Prevention*, July 2009.

Kim Painter, "New Scan for Skin Cancer Goes Full-Body Route," *USA Today*, July 1, 2008. www.usatoday.com/news/health/painter/2008-06-01-yourhealth_N.htm.

Alice Park, "Scalp, Neck Skin Cancer Most Lethal," *Time*, April 21, 2008. www.time.com/time/health/article/0,8599,1733719,00.htm.

Julie Rawe, "Why Teens Are Obsessed with Tanning," *Time*, July 31, 2006. www.time.com/time/magazine/article/0,9171,1220506,00.html.

Redbook, "5 Cancer Myths—Busted," Your Health, March 2009.

Adam Voiland, "The Indoor Tanning Industry Wants You," *U.S. News & World Report*, June 25, 2008. http://health.usnews.com.

———, "Why Skin Cancer Kills More Men than Women," *U.S. News & World Report*, June 26, 2008. http://health.usnews.com.

Sylvia Pagan Westphal, "High Hopes for a New Kind of Gene," *Smithsonian*, July 2009.

Internet Resources

AT-RISC, "Skin Cancer After Organ Transplantation: Prevention Is the Key," AT-RISC Alliance, 2009. http://at-risc.org/common/ATRISCfactsheet3.pdf.

Kevin Berman, "Skin Cancer, Medications and Medical Conditions," Skin Cancer Connection, June 8, 2009. www.healthcentral.com/skin-cancer/c/83/73956/skin-medications/pf.

Salynn Boyles, "WHO: Tanning Beds Cause Cancer," WebMD Health News, July 29, 2009. www.medscape.com/viewarticle/706726.

Jean Enersen, "A New Fast-Growing Skin Cancer to Watch Out For," King 5, March 11, 2009. www.king5.com/health/stories/NW_031109HEB-skin-cancer-LJ262031ff.html?rss.

Martha M. Grout, "Skin Cancer, Sun and Vitamin D," Arizona Center for Advanced Medicine, 2009. www.arizonaadvancedmedicine.com/articles/skin_cancer.html.

*Science*Daily, "New Genetic Culprit in Deadly Skin Cancer Revealed," September 1, 2009. www.sciencedaily.com/releases/2009/08/090831212427.htm.

INDEX